Essential Research for Evidence-Based Practice in Nursing Care

Mohammed Al Maqbali

Essential Research for Evidence-Based Practice in Nursing Care

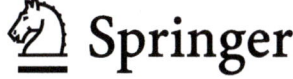 Springer

Mohammed Al Maqbali
Department of Nursing
Fatima College of Health Sciences
Al Ain, United Arab Emirates

ISBN 978-3-031-78297-8   ISBN 978-3-031-78298-5   (eBook)
https://doi.org/10.1007/978-3-031-78298-5

This Springer imprint is published by the registered company Springer Nature Switzerland AG
The registered company address is: Gewerbestrasse 11, 6330 Cham, Switzerland

If disposing of this product, please recycle the paper.

Preface

This textbook is designed to equip both novice and experienced nursing researchers with a comprehensive understanding of research methodologies and their application in clinical practice. With the increasing emphasis on evidence-based practice, this book covers a broad range of research strategies, ethical considerations, and practical examples that bridge the gap between theory and practice. By integrating current trends and emerging technologies, this textbook ensures that nurses are well-prepared to meet the evolving challenges of healthcare. Each chapter presents a detailed exploration of critical topics in nursing research, making it a valuable resource for nursing students, practitioners, and researchers alike.

Nursing research serves as a foundational pillar for advancing patient care and improving healthcare outcomes. Chapter 1 introduces the importance of nursing research in the modern healthcare landscape, tracing its historical evolution from Florence Nightingale's pioneering efforts to the current focus on evidence-based practice. This chapter provides a comprehensive overview of key research methodologies—quantitative, qualitative, and mixed methods—and highlights how nursing research drives innovation in healthcare. Readers will gain a deep understanding of how research enhances patient outcomes, supports healthcare decision-making, and contributes to professional development in nursing.

Quantitative research is essential in generating empirical data that informs nursing practice. Chapter 2 focuses on the principles and methodologies of quantitative research, including research design, sampling techniques, data collection methods, and statistical analysis. This chapter emphasizes the importance of objectivity and precision in conducting research that measures variables related to patient care, treatment outcomes, and healthcare interventions. By exploring experimental, non-experimental, and quasi-experimental designs, this chapter equips nurses with the tools necessary to conduct rigorous and reliable quantitative studies.

Qualitative research provides rich, detailed insights into patient experiences and healthcare interactions. Chapter 3 delves into qualitative methodologies such as phenomenology, grounded theory, and ethnography, which are critical for understanding complex healthcare phenomena. This chapter outlines flexible and adaptive data collection methods, including interviews, focus groups, and observations, which allow researchers to capture the nuanced narratives of patients and healthcare providers. By offering detailed guidance on data analysis and interpretation, this chapter empowers nurses to integrate qualitative research findings into practice to improve patient-centered care.

Mixed-methods research combines the strengths of both quantitative and qualitative approaches to offer a holistic understanding of complex research questions. Chapter 4 explores how mixed methods are particularly useful in addressing multifaceted healthcare challenges. This chapter discusses the philosophical foundations, such as pragmatism, that guide mixed-methods research, and presents detailed explanations of convergent, explanatory sequential, exploratory sequential, and embedded research designs. Nurses will learn how to integrate quantitative and qualitative data effectively to draw comprehensive conclusions that enhance the quality of nursing research.

Ethical considerations are paramount in conducting nursing research, particularly when human participants are involved. Chapter 5 provides a thorough examination of the ethical principles that guide nursing research, including beneficence, respect for human dignity, and justice. This chapter highlights the historical context of unethical research practices and their impact on the development of contemporary ethical standards. It also discusses the role of Institutional Review Boards (IRBs) in protecting participants' rights and ensuring that nursing research adheres to the highest ethical standards. This chapter ensures that readers are well-equipped to conduct ethically sound research.

Evidence-based practice (EBP) is the cornerstone of modern nursing care, and Chap. 6 focuses on the integration of research evidence into clinical practice. This chapter traces the development of EBP, from its origins in medicine to its current application in nursing. Readers will learn about the hierarchy of evidence, systematic appraisal of research, and the steps for translating evidence into practice. This chapter also reviews various EBP models and frameworks, such as the Iowa and Johns Hopkins models, offering practical guidance for their implementation in healthcare settings. This chapter emphasizes the importance of continuously updating clinical practice based on the latest and most reliable research to improve patient outcomes.

This textbook provides a comprehensive and in-depth guide to nursing research, covering a wide range of methodologies, ethical considerations, and practical applications. Whether you are a student embarking on your first research project or an experienced nurse seeking to refine your research skills, this book serves as a valuable resource. It equips nurses with the knowledge and tools necessary to conduct impactful research that enhances patient care, advances nursing practice, and contributes meaningfully to the healthcare profession.

Al Ain, United Arab Emirates   Mohammed Al Maqbali

Acknowledgments

The journey of completing this textbook has been both challenging and rewarding, and it would not have been possible without the support and encouragement of many individuals and organizations.

First and foremost, I would like to express my deep gratitude to my colleagues and collaborators, who have generously shared their knowledge and expertise throughout this process. Their contributions have been invaluable in shaping the content of this book and ensuring its relevance to the nursing profession. I am particularly grateful to *June Yasay*, Senior Officer Librarian, for her invaluable insights and support in providing access to essential library resources, books, and articles, which greatly enriched the quality of the chapters.

I would also like to extend my heartfelt thanks to the team at Springer for their unwavering support and guidance throughout this project. Their dedication to producing high-quality academic publications has been instrumental in bringing this textbook to completion. I am especially grateful for their professionalism and editorial expertise, particularly *Pinky Sathishkumar and Marie-Elia Come-Garry*, who ensured that the final product meets the highest standards of academic rigor.

Special thanks go to the nursing students, practitioners, and researchers, whose experiences and dedication to advancing patient care through evidence-based practice continue to inspire my work. Your commitment to improving healthcare is the driving force behind this book. Finally, I dedicate this book to nurses everywhere who, through their dedication and commitment to evidence-based practice, continue to transform healthcare for the better.

Contents

About the Author

Mohammed Al Maqbali , RN, Dip. Admin., BSc (Hons), MSc, PhD, AFHEA, MRSB is an Assistant Professor in the Department of Nursing at Fatima College of Health Sciences in Al Ain, UAE. With over 24 years of experience, including 20 years in clinical settings such as surgical and critical care, including the operating room, Dr. Al Maqbali brings a wealth of practical and academic expertise. His leadership roles in administration and management further complement his holistic approach to nursing education.

Recognized for his expertise in research methodologies and evidence-based practice, Dr. Al Maqbali focuses on guiding undergraduate students toward integrating research into clinical practice. His mentorship has shaped many students' understandings of the critical role research plays in improving healthcare outcomes.

Dr. Al Maqbali's extensive research portfolio includes publications in peer-reviewed journals and book chapters, covering quantitative and qualitative studies, systematic reviews, and meta-analyses. His work aims to advance nursing knowledge and apply research to enhance patient care. In addition to his academic role, Dr. Al Maqbali remains closely involved in clinical practice, bridging the gap between research, education, and real-world healthcare settings.

Introduction to Nursing Research

1

Learning Outcomes

By the end of this chapter, you will be able to:

1. Understand the historical evolution of nursing research from its origins with Florence Nightingale to its current role in modern healthcare.
2. Identify the importance of nursing research in enhancing patient care, improving healthcare systems, and advancing the nursing profession.
3. Differentiate between research methodologies—quantitative, qualitative, and mixed methods—and understand how each contributes to nursing knowledge and practice.
4. Formulate clear, focused, and relevant research questions that guide meaningful investigations in nursing.
5. Apply research findings to clinical practice, ensuring that nursing care is grounded in the most current and reliable evidence.
6. Recognize how engaging in research contributes to personal and professional growth, enhancing career opportunities and recognition in the healthcare field.

1.1 Introduction

Embarking on a nursing career in today's dynamic healthcare environment is both exhilarating and demanding. Nurses navigate their clinical duties in a scenario where the profession, coupled with the overarching healthcare infrastructure, necessitates a remarkable spectrum of skills and expertise from them. The expectation is that nurses deliver adept, premium care with compassion, all while adhering to cost-effectiveness principles. Achieving these multifaceted objective mandates that nurses constantly seek, assess, and assimilate new information, morphing it into actionable insights during clinical decision-making processes. In this modern era, it is imperative for nurses to embrace the journey of lifelong learning, cultivating the ability to reflect upon, evaluate, and adapt their clinical practices in light of burgeoning knowledge stemming from meticulous nursing and healthcare research.

1.2 Definition of Research

Research is a rigorous systematic inquiry or exploration that authenticates and refines prevailing knowledge while cultivating new understanding [1]. Rigorous systematic exploration implies structured planning, orderly organization, and sustained diligence. The overarching objective of research is to amass an empirical corpus of knowledge for a specific discipline or profession, like nursing.

The pinnacle aim of research is to sculpt, hone, and broaden the realm of knowledge. The trajectory of nurses increasingly intertwining with disciplined investigative pursuits is notable, casting positive ripples across the profession and the individuals it serves. **Nursing research** embodies a methodical quest aimed at forging reliable evidence concerning matters pivotal to the nursing domain, encapsulating nursing practice, education, administration, and informatics.

The primary aim of this book centers on nursing research and the application of evidence-based practice in nursing, providing a deep dive into rigorously conducted studies designed to direct nursing practice and improve the health and quality of life of the patients under nursing care. Nursing research often originates from questions sparked by challenges encountered in practice—challenges that might echo the reader's own experiences. By delving into a thorough exploration of real-world nursing quandaries and the research efforts to solve them, this book strives to narrow the chasm between research and practical application. It highlights the critical necessity of integrating evidence-based findings into daily nursing practice to promote better patient care outcomes and adeptly navigate the intricacies prevalent in today's healthcare milieu.

1.3   Importance of Nursing Research

The realm of healthcare is ever evolving, pivoting on the axis of relentless research and discovery. Nursing, a vital cog in this expansive mechanism, continually adapts through research to meet the burgeoning demands of patient care. Research serves as the backbone of healthcare advancements, with nursing research often being a cornerstone. It provides valuable insights into patient needs, care procedures, and the efficacy of healthcare systems. For instance, research by nurses on infection control has been pivotal in curbing hospital-acquired infections, thus elevating patient safety standards. Additionally, interdisciplinary research collaborations between nurses, doctors, and other healthcare professionals spawn innovative solutions to complex health-care quandaries, further propelling the sector forward.

At the heart of nursing is the unyielding commitment to exemplary patient care. Research in nursing is a linchpin for cultivating evidence-based practices that markedly improve patient outcomes. Through meticulous research, nurses develop, refine, and implement care protocols ensuring the patients receive the most effective care. For example, research on pain management has significantly ameliorated the quality of life for patients with chronic illnesses. Moreover, by identifying the determinants of patient satisfaction and areas of improvement, nursing research continually refines the patient care model, striving for excellence.

Professional development in nursing is intertwined with a culture of research. Nurses engaging in research not only contribute to the profession but also to their personal growth. Research nurtures a culture of continuous learning, fostering a proficient and knowledgeable workforce ready to tackle the evolving healthcare challenges. It also plays a seminal role in shaping nursing education, ensuring it remains relevant and robust in preparing the nurses of tomorrow. By partaking in research, nurses carve a niche for themselves in the healthcare ecosystem, enhancing their professional recognition and career progression.

However, nursing research is not without its set of challenges. Resource constraints, time limitations, and the need for advanced research skills often act as deterrents. Despite these hurdles, the trajectory of nursing research appears promising, buoyed by technological advancements and a burgeoning interest in multidisciplinary research.

Research in nursing is an indispensable tool for propelling healthcare forward, refining patient care, and fostering professional development. As nurses delve deeper into the realm of research, they unlock new dimensions of knowledge, contribute to a better understanding of patient care nuances, and play a crucial role in the advancement of healthcare. The sustenance and growth of nursing as a profession are inextricably linked to its research endeavors, reaffirming the indelible importance of research in nursing.

1. **Evidence-Based Practice:** Research helps in the development and implementation of evidence-based practice, ensuring that nursing care is based on the latest and most accurate information.
2. **Improving Patient Care:** Through research, nurses can find better ways of providing care, which can lead to improved patient outcomes, satisfaction, and overall experience.
3. **Healthcare Innovation:** Research in nursing contributes to innovation in healthcare, often leading to the development of new techniques, interventions, or medications.
4. **Professional Development:** Engaging in research can significantly contribute to a nurse's professional growth, enhancing their knowledge, skills, and career opportunities.
5. **Policy Development:** Nursing research can inform healthcare policy at both institutional and governmental levels, helping to shape regulations and standards of care.
6. **Cost Efficiency:** Research can help identify more cost-effective ways of delivering healthcare, which is crucial in the current era of budget constraints and rising healthcare costs.
7. **Education and Training:** Research contributes to nursing education by keeping the curriculum updated with the latest findings, ensuring that new nurses are well-prepared for the challenges of modern healthcare.
8. **Addressing Health Disparities:** Research can help address health disparities by identifying inequities in healthcare delivery and outcomes among different population groups.
9. **Interdisciplinary Collaboration:** Nursing research often involves collaboration with other healthcare professionals, promoting an interdisciplinary approach to healthcare challenges.
10. **Increasing the Visibility and Value of Nursing:** Through research, the critical role of nurses in healthcare delivery and outcomes is highlighted, which in turn increases the visibility and perceived value of nursing as a profession.
11. **Enhancing Quality of Life:** Research in areas like pain management, palliative care, and patient education helps in enhancing the quality of life for individuals, especially those with chronic illnesses or terminal conditions.
12. **Preparing for Future Healthcare Challenges:** Research in nursing helps in understanding and preparing for future healthcare challenges, be it emerging diseases, aging populations, or healthcare delivery in remote or underserved areas.

1.4   History of Nursing Research

Over the past 180 years, nursing research has experienced profound changes, beginning with its inception in the nineteenth century through the work of Florence Nightingale [2]. It is evident that nursing research did not consistently possess the level of influence and significance it currently holds. In fact, after Nightingale's pioneering contributions, there was a distinct lack of literature dedicated to nursing research in subsequent years. An exploration of nursing's history offers nurses a meaningful opportunity to gain a deeper understanding of their professional identity and how the past has left a lasting impact on the present.

Florence Nightingale, the pioneering nurse researcher in 1859, focused on the crucial role of creating a favorable environment for enhancing patients' physical and mental well-being [3]. Her investigations encompassed ventilation, cleanliness, water quality, and dietary choices, all aimed at understanding their impact on patients' health. Nightingale's research prowess extended to meticulous data collection and statistical analysis, notably during the Crimean War, where she studied soldiers' morbidity and mortality rates and their influencing factors, presenting her findings through tables and charts [4].

Nightingale's research initiatives had profound implications, leading the military to acknowledge the rights of the sick to receive adequate food, suitable accommodations, and appropriate medical care, resulting in a substantial reduction in mortality rates [5]. Her influence extended to society, which began to assume the responsibility of testing public water sources, improving sanitation, preventing starvation, and ultimately lowering morbidity and mortality rates [6].

Following Florence Nightingale's contributions, the nursing literature witnessed a prolonged period with limited research activity. This limited activity was attributed to the apprenticeship-based nature of nursing. The nature of nursing research that gradually emerged around the turn of the century closely mirrored the challenges faced by nurses. However, most of these studies were conducted from 1900 to 1940, focusing on nursing students' education. As the number of nurses who were educated at universities increased, the scope of these studies also became more extensive. The scope of nursing studies expanded during the 1940s due to the nursing workforce's increasing demand following the Second World War. During the 1950s, various factors combined to boost the research activity in the field. During the 1960s, some nursing leaders expressed their concerns about the lack of proper research in the profession. During this time, numerous professional nursing associations set forth research agendas, and research that focused on practical clinical matters began to surface in published works [7].

As the 1970s approached, an increasing number of nurses engaged in research endeavors, and the discourse around theoretical and contextual aspects of nursing research underscored the demand for additional channels of communication. Likewise, research proficiency among nurses in the USA saw significant enhancement during the 1970s [7]. This was primarily a result of the growing cohort of nurses attaining doctoral degrees, with the availability of fellowships playing a pivotal role in fostering the development of these research capabilities.

The 1980s marked a pivotal era in the development of nursing research. A surge in the number of qualified nurse researchers, the widespread availability of computers for data collection and analysis, and an increasing recognition of

research as an essential component of professional nursing prompted nursing leaders to address fresh challenges and considerations [8]. There was a greater emphasis on the nature of research questions, the methodologies employed for data collection and analysis, the integration of research with theoretical frameworks, and the application of research findings in practical nursing.

As the 1990s unfolded, nursing practice underwent a clinical transformation in response to societal, medical, scientific, and technological advancements. Changes in nursing practice began to emerge as a result of research-based practice guidelines, driven by collaborative efforts from individuals within and outside the nursing profession, all working to stimulate and support clinical nursing research [9].

From the twenty-first century, there was a notable transformation in nursing research. It transitioned from predominantly descriptive studies to encompass more explanatory and predictive methods, frequently combining qualitative and quantitative approaches [10]. Currently, nursing research adopts a multidisciplinary perspective, reflecting its increasing diversity and intricacy. The field of scientific investigation in nursing research has broadened to encompass clinical, healthcare system, and outcome-oriented research as well as studies related to education and administration.

1.5   Types of Research

The research knowledge required for practical application in nursing is both detailed and comprehensive, emphasizing a focus on processes and outcomes. To attain this knowledge, a diverse set of research methods is necessary. Three commonly utilized research methods for generating empirical knowledge in nursing practice include quantitative, qualitative, and mixed methods. These research approaches are vital for producing evidence that supports the objectives of the nursing profession.

Since the 1930s, most researchers have restricted the scope of their scientific methods to only quantitative research [11]. This type of research is rooted in positivism or logical empiricism. This philosophy helps develop scientific insight by allowing the researcher to maintain a non-interactive demeanor and avoid bias. This type of research is a formal process utilized to collect numerical data for a specific study. It involves examining the relationships among various factors and determining their causes and effects.

Conversely, qualitative research entails a systematic, in-depth, and subjective approach that aims to comprehend life experiences, social dynamics, and cultures from the perspectives of individuals involved. This notion is not a recent addition to behavioral and social sciences, as indicated by Glaser and Strauss in 1967 and Baumrind in 1980 [12, 13]. The goal of this research approach is to provide a deeper understanding of the human condition. It aims to explore the various factors that influence our lives.

The two types of research, qualitative and quantitative, are complementary as they provide different kinds of knowledge that can be useful in nursing practice Table 1.1. Understanding the difference between these two forms of research will help you critically appraise and identify their applications. Both of these require a lot of expertise and are prone to producing studies that are both thorough and demanding. The terms qualitative and quantitative are used to describe various research approaches. There are many factors that can help distinguish these two types of research. For instance, the design of data types and research questions can help distinguish them. In addition, an objective worldview is assumed in quantitative research. The goal of quantitative research is to collect empirical evidence, which is usually done through the use of observations that are measurable through five senses. This type of study often involves using numerical data to test hypotheses, and it also challenges objectivity. On the other, qualitative research is focused on the recognition of the world's subjectivity. This discipline acknowledges various realities that exist in different contexts and over time. Qualitative research aims to provide a deeper understanding of human behaviors by examining verbal descriptions.

Another crucial aspect of quantitative and qualitative approaches is the association with two distinct styles of reasoning. Deductive reasoning, primarily aligned with quantitative research, follows a path from the general to the specific. In this approach, researchers utilize theories to logically derive hypotheses. On the other hand, inductive reasoning, commonly linked with qualitative approaches, follows a trajectory from the specific to the general. Researchers employing inductive reasoning extrapolate general insights from specific instances, allowing them to con-

Table 1.1 Characteristic of Quantitative and Qualitative Research

Characteristic	Quantitative	Qualitative
Focuses	Emphasizes breadth, seeking patterns and generalizability	Emphasizes depth, exploring meanings and contextual understanding
Reality	Assumes an objective reality that can be measured and quantified	Acknowledges multiple subjective realities, context-dependent
Reasoning approach	**Deductive** reasoning, moving from the general to the specific	**Inductive** reasoning, moving from the specific to the general
Number of participants	Large and representative samples for generalizability	Small, purposive samples to explore in-depth insights within context
Concept of participant	Participants are seen as data sources, often with anonymized identities	Participants are active co-creators of meaning; their perspectives are crucial
Data type	Numerical and standardized data	Non-numerical, textual, context-dependent data
Data collection	Structured methods like surveys, experiments, and measurements	Unstructured methods like interviews, observations, and open-ended surveys
Analysis type	Statistical analysis involves numerical computations	Qualitative analysis, involves thematic coding, content analysis, narrative exploration

struct an overall summary of the phenomenon under investigation [1].

Mixed methods research is an investigative approach that melds quantitative and qualitative research methodologies within a single study. The research objectives and questions are formulated to encompass both the quantitative and qualitative aspects of the investigation. Depending on the study's purpose, researchers may lean more toward either a quantitative or qualitative research method. Typically, mixed methods studies involve gathering both types of data—qualitative and quantitative—and analyzing them as per the study's design [14]. The integration and analysis of data are carried out according to the study's specifications. There are instances where quantitative and qualitative research methods are applied concurrently or sequentially, guided by the desired knowledge outcomes.

1.6   Formulating the Research Question

Formulating a research question is a pivotal and initial step in the research process, serving as the compass that guides the entire study. A well-crafted research question not only delineates the scope of investigation but also lays the foundation for meaningful inquiry. This process involves a systematic approach that incorporates various considerations to ensure clarity, specificity, and relevance.

At its core, the development of a research question involves navigating through a series of steps designed to refine a broad topic into a focused and answerable query. This journey begins with the identification of a general area of interest and extends to a comprehensive review of existing literature, ensuring that the proposed question is both novel and contributes to the existing body of knowledge. The researcher must balance specificity with feasibility, aiming to create a question that is not only clear in its intent but also practical to address within the given resources and constraints.

Whether quantitative, qualitative, or a blend of both methodologies, the type of research dictates the formulation process. Quantitative research

often leans toward deductive reasoning, moving from general theories to specific hypotheses, while qualitative research embraces inductive reasoning, allowing for the emergence of patterns and insights from specific instances.

Throughout this developmental journey, the researcher is prompted to refine their focus, articulate the purpose of the study, and consider the relevance of the research question to the broader academic or professional landscape. Seeking feedback from peers, mentors, or advisors becomes an integral aspect, providing valuable insights that contribute to the question's enhancement.

As researchers navigate these steps, they must remain conscious of potential biases, ensuring that the question is framed objectively to yield unbiased results. Additionally, the question should be dynamic, allowing for potential revisions as the research progresses and new insights emerge.

In essence, the art of formulating a research question is an intricate dance between curiosity, existing knowledge, and methodological considerations. It is an intellectual endeavor that sets the stage for a meaningful exploration, inviting researchers to embark on a journey of discovery and contribute substantively to their field of study.

1.6.1   Identify a Topic

Identifying a broad research topic serves as the cornerstone for the entire research process, akin to selecting the initial coordinates on a map. In this crucial step, researchers navigate the vast landscape of potential subjects within their field, contemplating overarching themes that resonate with their interests and the broader academic or professional context. For instance, a nursing researcher might initially explore broad areas such as patient care, healthcare technologies, or nursing education.

This exploration sets the stage for a comprehensive literature review, where researchers delve into existing studies to discern the current state of knowledge and pinpoint potential research gaps. Refining the broad topic requires a delicate balance, seeking a focus that is both novel and contributes meaningfully to the existing body of knowledge.

The choice of research methodology, whether quantitative, qualitative, or a blend of both, plays a pivotal role in shaping the formulation process. This initial step involves transitioning from a broad area of interest to a more refined focus, guided by the researcher's discernment and the quest for clear, specific, and purposeful inquiry.

Seeking a balance between specificity and feasibility, researchers embark on a journey that prompts them to articulate the relevance of their research question to the broader academic or professional landscape. Feedback from peers, mentors, or advisors enriches the process, ensuring diverse perspectives contribute to the question's enhancement. In essence, identifying a broad topic is the opening act in the research narrative, setting the trajectory for a focused and impactful exploration.

The initiation of the research process hinges on the pivotal step of identifying a topic that not only captivates the researcher's interest but also aligns with the broader context of their academic or professional domain. Selecting an appropriate topic is akin to choosing the North Star, providing direction and purpose for the entire research endeavor.

At the genesis of this journey, researchers are encouraged to cast a wide net, exploring diverse areas within their field to identify a general area of interest. For instance, a nursing researcher may start by contemplating overarching themes such as patient care, healthcare technologies, or nursing education.

1.6.2 Conduct a Literature Review

Once a broad topic is identified, the next crucial step in the research journey is to conduct a comprehensive literature review. This phase is akin to exploring a vast library of knowledge, where researchers immerse themselves in existing studies and scholarly works related to their chosen field.

The primary goal of the literature review is twofold: to understand the current landscape of knowledge and to identify gaps or areas where further exploration is warranted. Researchers delve into academic journals, books, conference proceedings, and other reputable sources to grasp the state of affairs in their chosen domain. For instance, a nursing researcher focusing on patient-centered care might examine studies on communication strategies, holistic nursing practices, and patient outcomes.

By synthesizing existing research, researchers gain insights into established theories, methodologies, and findings. They identify key themes, controversies, and unanswered questions that shape the trajectory of their own study. This process not only informs the researcher but also ensures that the proposed research question is not redundant but contributes meaningfully to the existing body of knowledge.

Moreover, a well-conducted literature review provides a theoretical framework for the research, helping researchers situate their work within the broader academic discourse. It establishes the context for the study, clarifying the rationale behind the chosen research question and methodology.

In navigating this scholarly landscape, researchers must critically evaluate the reliability and validity of the sources they consult. Assessing the methodology, sample size, and findings of existing studies ensures that the literature review is grounded in rigorous scholarship.

Conducting a literature review is, therefore, a meticulous and intellectual endeavor that guides researchers from the broad landscape of a chosen topic to a nuanced understanding of the current state of knowledge. It serves as the intellectual foundation upon which the research question is refined, ensuring that the subsequent inquiry is both informed and purposeful.

1.6.3 Narrow Down Your Focus

Having immersed oneself in the existing body of knowledge, the next pivotal step in crafting a research question is to narrow down the focus. This stage is analogous to zooming in on a specific area within the broader landscape identified during the literature review.

Researchers' transition from a panoramic view to a more detailed examination, refining their initial broad topic based on the insights gained from the literature. This refinement is guided by the recognition of patterns, gaps, or specific aspects within the literature that warrant further exploration. For instance, a nursing researcher exploring patient-centered care might narrow the focus to a particular aspect, such as the impact of communication strategies on patient satisfaction.

The aim is to strike a balance between specificity and generality, ensuring that the research question is focused enough to yield meaningful insights while remaining broad enough to encapsulate various facets of the chosen theme. This narrowing down process is crucial for formulating a question that is not only answerable but also aligns with the researcher's goals and available resources.

Moreover, this stage prompts researchers to consider the feasibility of their chosen focus. They must assess whether the scope of the research question is manageable within the constraints of time, resources, and ethical considerations. Refining the focus at this juncture ensures that the research remains practical and achievable.

The transition from a broad topic to a narrowed focus is an iterative process, involving reflection, consultation with peers or mentors, and a continuous reevaluation of the research goals. It represents a critical juncture where the researcher defines the specific territory they will explore, laying the groundwork for the subsequent articulation of a clear and purposeful research question.

1.6.4 Define the Purpose of Your Study

With a narrowed focus in sight, the next crucial step in formulating a research question is to explicitly define the purpose of the study. This stage is akin to setting the compass for the research journey, articulating the overarching goal or objective that the researcher aims to accomplish.

The purpose of the study provides a clear direction and rationale for the research question. It answers the fundamental question: "Why is this research important, and what do I hope to achieve?" For example, a nursing researcher narrowing down the focus to communication strategies in patient-centered care might define the purpose as understanding how effective communication impacts patient satisfaction and healthcare outcomes [15].

This definition of purpose serves as a guiding beacon, ensuring that every aspect of the research, from the formulation of the question to the collection and analysis of data, aligns with the overarching goal. It establishes the context for the research, outlining the specific contribution study aims to make to the existing body of knowledge.

Moreover, the purpose statement sets the tone for the entire research endeavor. It influences the choice of research methodology, the selection of variables, and the framing of hypotheses or research questions. Whether the study aims to explore, describe, explain, predict, or evaluate, defining the purpose provides clarity on the intended outcome.

In essence, defining the purpose of the study is a pivotal act of intentionality in the research process. It transforms the research question from a curious inquiry into a purposeful pursuit, laying the foundation for a study that is not only academically rigorous but also deeply meaningful in its contribution to the chosen field.

1.6.5 Consider the Type of Research

Once the purpose of the study is clearly defined, the researcher must make a pivotal decision regarding the type of research to be conducted. This decision influences the entire research design and methodology. Research can broadly be categorized into quantitative, qualitative, or a combination of both, known as mixed methods.

1.6.5.1 Quantitative Research

In quantitative research, the emphasis is on collecting numerical data and employing statistical analyses to draw conclusions. This approach is characterized by structured methodologies, surveys, experiments, and a focus on measurable variables. For instance, a quantitative study in nursing might involve assessing the effectiveness of a specific medication on patient recovery rates.

1.6.5.2 Qualitative Research

Qualitative research, on the other hand, is exploratory and seeks to understand the underlying motivations, attitudes, and behaviors of individuals. It often involves unstructured or semi-structured methods such as interviews, observations, or content analysis. In nursing, a qualitative study could delve into the lived experiences of nurses caring for patients in challenging environments.

1.6.5.3 Mixed Methods Research

Mixed methods research integrates both quantitative and qualitative approaches in a single study. Researchers using mixed methods aim to gain a comprehensive understanding by combining numerical data with in-depth explorations. For instance, in nursing research, a mixed methods study might involve collecting survey data on patient satisfaction (quantitative) and conducting interviews to understand the nuances of their experiences (qualitative).

The choice between these approaches depends on the nature of the research question, the researcher's philosophical stance, and the depth of understanding sought. Quantitative methods are well-suited for testing hypotheses and identifying patterns, while qualitative methods excel in exploring complex phenomena and providing context-rich insights. Mixed methods, as the name suggests, offer the benefits of both approaches.

Considering the type of research is a critical juncture that shapes subsequent decisions, including data collection methods, sampling strategies, and the overall structure of the study. It aligns the research approach with the research-er's goals, ensuring that the chosen methodology is the most effective means to answer the research question.

1.6.6 Ask Clear and Specific Questions

Having navigated through the foundational steps, the researcher now focuses on the pivotal task of crafting clear and specific research questions. These questions serve as the compass, guiding the study's trajectory and determining the nature of the investigation. Clarity and specificity are paramount, ensuring that the research questions are focused, answerable, and aligned with the study's purpose.

1.6.6.1 Clarity of Language

Express the research questions in clear and straightforward language. Ambiguity can lead to confusion and hinder the precision required in the research process. For example, in nursing research, a clear question could be, "How does the implementation of a specific training program impact nurses' ability to communicate effectively with patients?"

Specificity in Scope

Refine the scope of the questions to avoid being overly broad or vague. Specificity ensures that the study remains manageable, and the research questions are tailored to the nuances of the chosen topic. For instance, a more specific question might be, "What communication strategies are most effective in improving patient understanding of post-operative care instructions?"

1.6.6.2 Alignment with Purpose

Ensure that the research questions directly align with the purpose of the study. Each question should contribute meaningfully to addressing the overarching goal, whether it is to explore, describe, explain, predict, or evaluate. This alignment provides a clear roadmap for the research. In the nursing example, the questions should directly relate to improving communication in healthcare settings.

1.6.6.3 Avoiding Assumptions

Craft questions that avoid assumptions and biases by ensuring the wording is neutral and objective. This approach allows for an unbiased exploration of the topic. For example, instead of presuming a positive impact, a question could be framed as, 'What factors influence nurses' perceptions of the effectiveness of the new communication training program?

1.6.6.4 Testability and Measurability

Formulate questions that are testable and measurable. This is particularly crucial in quantitative research where data must be collected and analyzed quantitatively. For qualitative research, clarity in the exploration of concepts and experiences is equally important.

Asking clear and specific questions is a skill that requires precision in language and a deep understanding of the research goals. These questions become the foundation for the subsequent stages of data collection, analysis, and interpretation, guiding the researcher toward meaningful insights and contributing to the scholarly conversation in their field.

1.6.7   Seek Feedback and Revise

After formulating clear and specific research questions, the next imperative step is to seek feedback from peers, mentors, or advisors. This collaborative process not only enriches the research endeavor but also ensures that the questions are refined to meet the highest standards of clarity, relevance, and scholarly rigor.

1.6.7.1 Peer Review

Share the formulated research questions with colleagues or peers who possess expertise in the field. Constructive feedback from diverse perspectives can reveal insights, potential biases, or overlooked aspects that contribute to refining the questions. This collaborative approach enhances the robustness of the research.

1.6.7.2 Mentor or Advisor Input

Seek guidance from mentors or advisors who have experience in the research domain. Their seasoned insights can provide invaluable suggestions for improving the questions, aligning them with the study's purpose, and ensuring that the methodology chosen is apt for the research goals.

1.6.7.3 Clarity and Precision

Request feedback on the clarity and precision of the questions. Ensure that the language used is accessible to a broader audience and that the questions precisely convey the intended meaning. Clarity is essential for effective communication and understanding.

1.6.7.4 Alignment with Goals

Confirm that the research questions align seamlessly with the overarching goals of the study. Feedback should address whether the questions contribute meaningfully to the purpose of the research and whether any adjustments are necessary for a more focused inquiry.

1.6.7.5 Feasibility and Practicality

Assess the feasibility and practicality of the research questions. Feedback can shed light on whether the questions are realistically answerable within the available resources, time frame, and ethical considerations. This pragmatic evaluation is crucial for the successful execution of the study.

1.6.7.6 Refinement and Iteration

Embrace the feedback received and be prepared to revise the research questions accordingly. The process of refinement is often iterative, involving multiple rounds of feedback and adjustment. Each iteration brings the questions closer to an optimal formulation that meets scholarly standards.

1.6.7.7 Consider Ethical Implications

Seek feedback on the ethical implications of the research questions. Ensure that the questions respect the rights and well-being of participants and adhere to ethical guidelines. This consideration is fundamental in maintaining the integrity of the research process.

Seeking feedback and revising the research questions is not merely a procedural step; it is an essential part of the scholarly dialogue. This collaborative approach fosters a culture of continuous improvement, ensuring that the research questions are robust, ethically sound, and poised to yield meaningful contributions to the chosen field of study.

References

1. Grove SK, Gray JR. Understanding nursing research: building an evidence-based practice. Amsterdam: Elsevier; 2022.
2. Schmidt NA, Brown JM. Evidence-based practice for nurses: appraisal and application of research. 4th ed. Burlington: Jones & Bartlett Learning; 2024.
3. Nightingale F. Notes on nursing: what it is, and what it is not. New York: D. Appleton; 1860.
4. Austin AL. The historical method in nursing. Nurs Res. 1958;7:4.
5. Moule P, Aveyard H, Goodman M. Nursing research: an introduction. London: SAGE; 2017.
6. Abel-Smith B. A history of the nursing profession. London: Heinemann; 1960.
7. Lewenson S, McAllister A. History of nursing education in the United States. In: Routledge international handbook of nurse education. 1st ed. New York: Routledge; 2020. p. 420.
8. Holt J. Whither nursing philosophy: past, present and future. Nurs Philos. 2023;24:e12442. https://doi.org/10.1111/nup.12442.
9. Skeen K, Wall BM. Nursing and eugenics in the early 20th century United States. Nurs Outlook. 2023;71:102018. https://doi.org/10.1016/j.outlook.2023.102018.
10. Tappen RM. Advanced nursing research: from theory to practice: from theory to practice. 3rd ed. Burlington: Jones & Bartlett Learning; 2022.
11. Boswell C, Cannon S. Introduction to nursing research: incorporating evidence-based practice. Burlington: Jones & Bartlett Learning; 2023.
12. Baumrind D. New directions in socialization research. Am Psychol. 1980;35:639–52. https://doi.org/10.1037/0003-066X.35.7.639.
13. Glaser BG, Strauss AL. The discovery of grounded theory: strategies for qualitative research. Venice: Aldine; 1967.
14. Creswell JW, Creswell JD. Research design: qualitative, quantitative, and mixed methods approaches. 6th ed. Los Angeles: SAGE; 2022.
15. Polit D, Beck C. Essentials of nursing research: appraising evidence for nursing practice. 10th ed. Philadelphia: LWW; 2021.

Quantitative Nursing Research

2

Learning Outcomes

By the end of this chapter, you will be able to:

1. Understand the principles and significance of quantitative research in nursing.
2. Differentiate between various quantitative research designs, including experimental, non-experimental, and quasi-experimental.
3. Apply appropriate sampling strategies to ensure the representativeness and validity of research studies.
4. Utilize statistical analysis techniques to interpret data and draw meaningful conclusions in nursing research.
5. Recognize the ethical considerations and challenges associated with conducting quantitative research in healthcare.
6. Integrate empirical evidence from quantitative research into clinical practice to enhance patient care and outcomes.

2.1 Introduction

Quantitative research is a multifaceted methodological approach dedicated to the systematic exploration of social phenomena through the utilization of statistical or numerical data [1]. This research paradigm relies on the premise that the phenomena under investigation can be accurately and meaningfully measured. Its overarching objective is to analyze data systematically, identi-

fying trends and relationships while validating the measurements acquired.

In the realm of nursing research, quantitative methodologies play a crucial role in providing empirical evidence and contributing to the development of evidence-based practices. Nurses and healthcare professionals often employ quantitative research to investigate various aspects of patient care, treatment outcomes, and healthcare interventions. This chapter aims to elucidate the foundational principles that underpin quantitative research in the context of nursing, emphasizing its significance in advancing the field.

One hallmark of quantitative research is its commitment to objectivity and the rigorous application of standardized measurement tools. Researchers meticulously design studies, ensuring that data collection methods are precise and reliable. Through the lens of quantitative inquiry, this chapter will explore the intricacies of designing and implementing studies in nursing research, addressing the challenges and nuances unique to the healthcare domain.

Furthermore, this chapter will delve into the statistical analyses' integral to quantitative research, unraveling the complexities of interpreting numerical data in the context of nursing studies. Understanding statistical methods is paramount for researchers and practitioners alike, as it empowers them to draw meaningful conclusions from the data and make informed decisions that directly impact patient care and healthcare policies.

In essence, this chapter serves as a comprehensive guide for nursing researchers seeking to engage with quantitative methodologies. By navigating through the fundamental concepts, methodologies, and statistical analyses, readers will gain a nuanced understanding of how quantitative research contributes to the advancement of nursing knowledge and practice.

Quantitative research methods involve the systematic empirical investigation through the collection, analysis, and interpretation of numerical data [2]. The primary aim of quantitative research is to quantify variables and establish statistical relationships, allowing researchers to draw objective conclusions and make generalizations about a population or phenomenon. This approach relies on structured research designs, standardized measurement tools, and statistical techniques to examine patterns, trends, and associations in data. The overarching goal of quantitative research is to provide a rigorous and quantifiable understanding of the studied phenomena, addressing questions related to "how much," "how many," or "to what extent," and thereby contributing valuable insights to the broader body of knowledge.

2.2   Design

Quantitative research designs employ systematic and objective approaches to generate and refine knowledge, primarily employing deductive reasoning and generalization [3]. Deductive reasoning involves initiating the research process with an established theory or framework, where concepts are already reduced into variables. The researcher then collects evidence to assess or test whether the theory or framework is substantiated. Generalization, on the other hand, refers to the extent to which conclusions drawn from evidence obtained from a sample can be extrapolated to the larger population.

In the domain of quantitative research, the primary emphasis is on quantifying the relationships between variables, specifically focusing on the independent or predictor variable and the dependent or outcome variable. These research designs fall broadly into two categories: non-experimental and experimental [4].

Non-experimental designs are utilized to depict, distinguish, or explore associations among variables, groups, or situations without directly manipulating them. Unlike experimental designs, non-experimental approaches do not incorporate random assignment, control groups, or the deliberate manipulation of variables. Instead, they rely solely on observational methods to identify patterns and relationships. Common examples of non-experimental designs include descriptive studies, which aim to portray characteristics or phenomena, and correlational studies, which investigate the degree of association between variables (Fig. 2.1).

This distinction between non-experimental and experimental designs highlights the versatility of quantitative research methodologies, providing researchers with a range of approaches to address diverse research questions and objectives within their specific areas of investigation.

2.2.1   Non-experimental

In non-experimental research, there is no manipulation of an independent variable, no need for a control group, and no random group assignments, distinguishing it from experimental and quasi-experimental designs [5]. Another term often used for this research type is "observational," highlighting the researcher's role in observing natural occurrences without intervening. Numerous non-experimental research designs exist, each typically classified based on its purpose (whether to describe, predict, or explain) and the temporal aspect (prospective—pertaining to the future, retrospective—pertaining to the past, or longitudinal—over time). The selection of a research design is determined by the intended goal of the research question, whether it aims to describe, predict, or explain the variable in question.

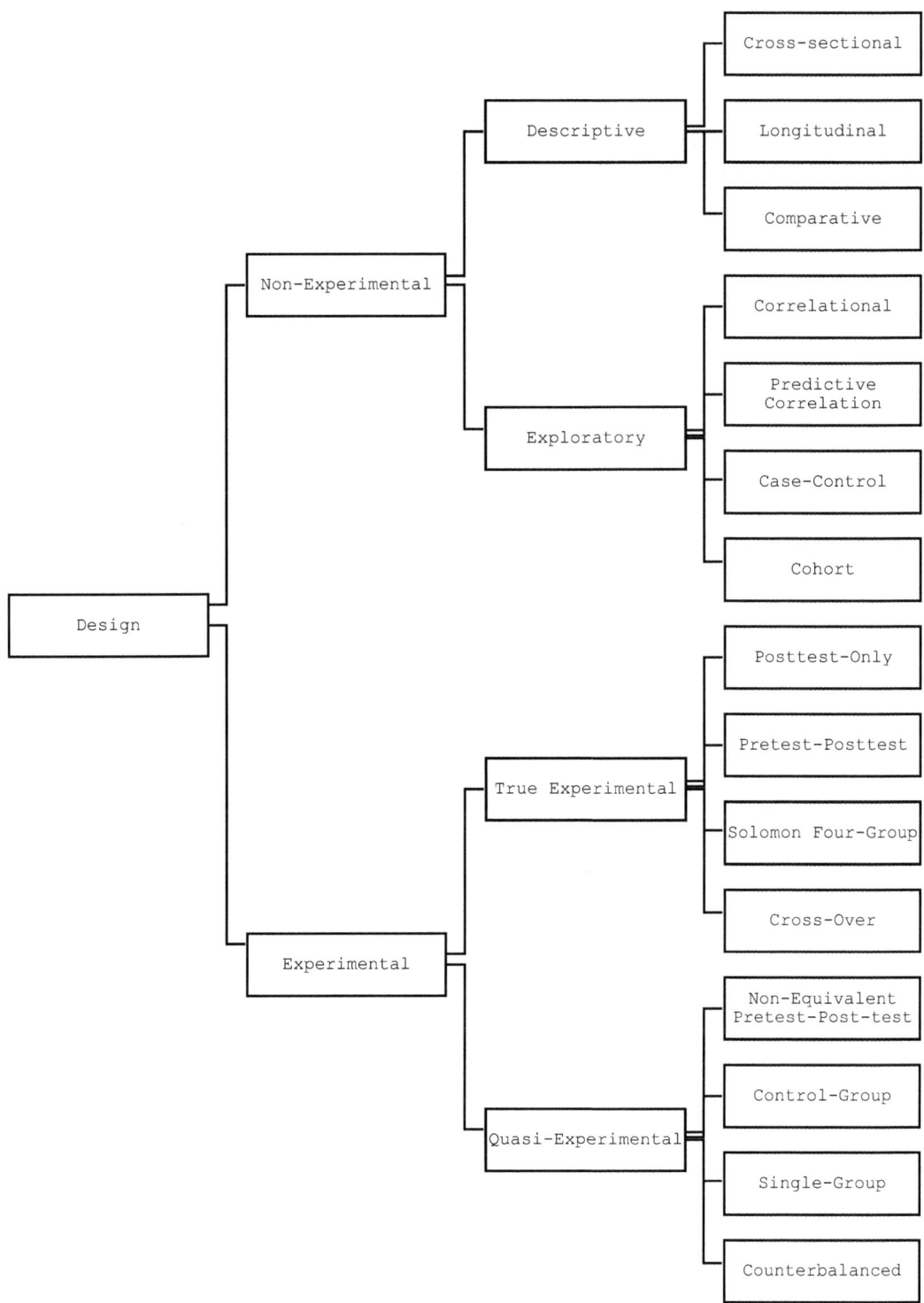

Fig. 2.1 Type of study designs

2.2.1.1 Descriptive Research

Descriptive research aims to depict the characteristics, behaviors, and conditions of individuals and groups [6]. This type of research can take on a retrospective, prospective, or longitudinal approach. Typically, a descriptive study focuses on a single sample. Surveys are commonly employed in descriptive research to offer an overall perspective on a group's characteristics. Researchers must identify variables of interest and determine the measurement methods for these variables. For instance, if researchers want to describe the fatigue levels experienced by nurses after night shifts, conducting this retrospectively may be challenging unless nurses have been documenting their experiences. Alternatively, researchers could opt for a *cross-sectional* study, observing a sample of nurses after specific night shifts and asking them to provide generalizations about their fatigue levels. Another option is a *longitudinal study*, involving nurses journaling their fatigue levels over an extended period. Alternatively, a prospective observation of fatigue behaviors in nurses after night shifts would entail real-time observations. Each of these designs constitutes a typical descriptive study, aiding researchers in describing fatigue levels within the sampled group of nurses.

Alternatively, researchers might undertake a *comparative* descriptive study with the aim of comparing groups and identifying naturally occurring differences. In this scenario, researchers could survey nurses about both their fatigue levels and any history of medication errors during night shifts. The naturally occurring samples would include nurses who have made errors and those who have not, allowing researchers to compare fatigue levels between the two groups. It is crucial to emphasize that the sole purpose of this approach is to describe fatigue levels and draw comparisons between groups. This research design does not permit drawing conclusions about a causal relationship between fatigue after night shifts and medication errors during the shifts. However, the findings of this descriptive study may provide a foundation for a future experimental study, such as a randomized controlled trial, to investigate the cause-and-effect relationship between fatigue after night shifts and medication errors specifically during the night shift.

2.2.1.2 Exploratory Research

Exploratory research constitutes a form of observational inquiry aimed at examining the connections between two or more variables. When researchers possess a hypothesis, they wish to test, they can employ an exploratory design. These studies may take on retrospective, prospective, or longitudinal formats, and various exploratory research designs exist, including correlational, predictive correlational, case-control, and cohort studies [1].

Correlational studies endeavor to gauge the extent of association among variables—whether they increase or decrease concurrently, move in opposite directions, or exhibit no connection. For instance, researchers might investigate the link between the workload of nurses and the occurrence of medication errors. This exploration could be retrospective with available workload data, but more likely requires a prospective or longitudinal approach. Researchers ultimately determine whether a relationship exists between workload and medication errors and elucidate the strength of that relationship. For instance, it may be revealed that as workload decreases, medication errors also decrease—a demonstration of an inverse relationship. However, inferring that reducing workload decreases a nurse's error risk would be erroneous. Other variables, such as the nurse's experience, might better explain this relationship. The link between workload and medication errors might be influenced by factors like experienced nurses predominantly working in high workload situations, making the correlation not a direct consequence of workload.

Predictive correlation studies resemble correlational studies but consider multiple independent variables to construct a model for anticipating when a particular outcome is probable. For instance, researchers aiming to predict medication errors may consider workload, nurse experience, education level, patient acuity, and patient ratios. Utilizing regression analysis, the statistical technique calculates the probability of a nurse committing an error based on these independent variables and identifies which variables contribute most significantly to the error risk.

Case-control research involves identifying a case (individual with the condition) and comparing it with a control (individual without the condition). This retrospective design involves looking back to gather data about factors that may have predisposed the case to the condition. Although not commonly used for exploring medication errors, the researcher could identify nurses who made errors (cases) and those who did not (controls). Subsequently, data from documents, interviews, and questionnaires would be collected to discern differences between the groups that might have influenced their risk for medication errors.

Cohort studies track a group of individuals over time, observing those who do not initially exhibit the outcome of interest to identify who will develop the outcome or disorder. Cohort studies often focus on how specific exposures affect the risk of developing a particular outcome. While exploring a relationship between workload and medication errors may not be suitable for a cohort study, changing the research question to investigate the association between bullying and medication errors related to workload could work. In this scenario, researchers might identify a cohort of new graduate nurses who have not experienced bullying related to workload. Over time, they collect data on medication errors and experiences of being bullied related to workload to determine if those exposed to bullying related to workload are more or less likely to make medication errors. While cohort studies cannot establish cause and effect, they can establish a time sequence and provide relative risk based on exposure, offering stronger evidence for causality than other observational designs.

2.2.2 Experimental

Experimental designs typically incorporate random assignment, the manipulation of independent variables, and stringent controls, enhancing the confidence in establishing cause-and-effect relationships [7]. The characteristic of random assignment ensures that each subject has an equal chance of being assigned to either the control or experimental group, aiming to eliminate systematic bias. It is important to note the distinction between random assignment and random sampling; while random sampling grants each subject an equal chance of being selected from a larger group for study participation, random assignment is a crucial element that sets true-experimental designs apart. To be classified as a true experiment, the design must encompass randomization, a control group, and the manipulation of a variable when exploring direct causal or predicted relationships between variables. Failure to meet any of these requirements results in the design being categorized as quasi-experimental. Researchers typically formulate level III research questions within the framework of true-experimental designs.

2.2.2.1 True Experimental

True-experimental designs systematically investigate cause-and-effect relationships between independent (predictor) and dependent (outcome) variables within highly controlled conditions. Among the simplest of these designs is the posttest-only control group design, and other common true-experimental designs encompass the pretest–posttest control group design, Solomon four-group design, and cross-over design [8].

In the *posttest-only* control group design, subjects are randomly assigned (R) to either a control or an experimental group, with no pretesting conducted. Following this, one group is exposed to a treatment (X) or a series of different treatments (X1, X2), and both groups undergo posttesting (O). This design allows researchers to meticulously examine the impact of the treatment or treatments on the dependent variables, providing valuable insights into the causal relationships under scrutiny.

Scenario: Investigating the Impact of a Training Program on Nursing Documentation Accuracy

In this study, nurses from a hospital are randomly assigned to either a control group or an experimental group. The control group continues with their regular documentation practices, while the experimental group undergoes a specialized training program focused on improving documentation accuracy.

Group Assignment:

Control Group: Nurses who continue with standard documentation practices.

Experimental Group: Nurses who receive the specialized training program.

Intervention:

Control Group: No additional intervention; they maintain their usual documentation routines.

Experimental Group: Receives a training program emphasizing best practices and strategies to enhance documentation accuracy.

Posttesting:

Both groups are then evaluated on their documentation accuracy through posttesting measures.

The posttest-only control group design in this nursing context allows researchers to assess whether the specialized training program has a discernible impact on the accuracy of nursing documentation when compared to the control group. By randomly assigning participants and conducting posttesting without pretesting, the study aims to draw conclusions about the effectiveness of the training program in improving documentation practices.

In the *pretest–posttest* control group design, often referred to as the classic experiment, subjects undergo random assignment (R) to either a control or experimental group. Both groups undergo pretesting (O). Following the pretest phase, the experimental group is subjected to a treatment (X) or a series of different treatments (X1, X2), and subsequently, both groups undergo posttesting (O). This design allows researchers to assess the impact of the treatment or treatments on the dependent variables while accounting for the initial differences identified during the pretest phase.

Scenario: Assessing the Effect of a Stress Reduction Intervention on Nursing Job Satisfaction

In this study, nurses from a healthcare facility are interested in examining the impact of a stress reduction intervention on job satisfaction. The researchers employ a pretest–posttest control group design to explore changes in job satisfaction levels before and after the intervention.

Group Assignment:

Control Group: Nurses assigned to this group undergo pretesting to establish their initial levels of job satisfaction. They continue with their regular work routine during the study period.

Experimental Group: Nurses assigned to this group also undergo pretesting to determine their initial levels of job satisfaction. However, they participate in a stress reduction intervention designed to enhance overall well-being.

Intervention:

Control Group: No specific stress reduction intervention; participants follow standard work routines.

Experimental Group: Participates in a stress reduction program designed to alleviate workplace stressors and improve overall well-being.

Pretesting:
Both groups are assessed for their baseline levels of job satisfaction before the intervention.

Intervention Implementation:
Experimental group participants undergo the stress reduction intervention.

Posttesting:
Both groups are then reassessed for job satisfaction after the intervention period.

By employing a pretest–posttest control group design, the study aims to compare changes in job satisfaction between the control and experimental groups, providing insights into the potential impact of the stress reduction intervention on nursing job satisfaction.

In the *Solomon four-group design*, subjects undergo random assignment (R) to one of four distinct groups. Two of these groups undergo pretesting (O), while the remaining two do not. Subsequently, only one pretested group and one non-pretested group are exposed to a treatment (X). Posttesting (O) is conducted for all groups to evaluate the effects of the treatment on the dependent variables. This design allows researchers to account for the potential impact of pretesting on the experimental outcomes, offering a more comprehensive understanding of the treatment's effects.

Scenario: Investigating the Impact of a New Patient Care Protocol on Nurse Performance
In this study, nurses are interested in assessing the effectiveness of a new patient care protocol on overall nurse performance. The researchers employ the Solomon Four-Group Design to account for potential interactions between pretesting and the intervention.

Group Assignment:
Group 1 (Pretested and Exposed to Intervention):
 – Pretested to measure baseline nurse performance.
 – Exposed to the new patient care protocol.
Group 2 (Pretested but Not Exposed to Intervention):
 – Pretested to measure baseline nurse performance.
 – Not exposed to the new patient care protocol.
Group 3 (Not Pretested but Exposed to Intervention):
 – Not pretested for baseline performance.
 – Exposed to the new patient care protocol.
Group 4 (Not Pretested and Not Exposed to Intervention):
 – Not pretested for baseline performance.
 – Not exposed to the new patient care protocol.

Intervention:
Groups 1 and 3 are exposed to the new patient care protocol.

Pretesting:
Groups 1 and 2 are pretested to measure baseline nurse performance.

Implementation of Intervention:
Groups 1 and 3 are exposed to the new patient care protocol.

Posttesting:
All groups are posttested to measure nurse performance after the intervention.

By employing the Solomon Four-Group Design, the study aims to not only assess the impact of the new patient care protocol but also consider potential interactions between pretesting and the intervention, providing a more comprehensive understanding of the intervention's effects on nurse performance.

In the *cross-over*, also known as counterbalanced, switchover, or rotation design, subjects are exposed to two treatments: one being the experimental treatment (XE) and the other a control or reference treatment (XC). Subjects are randomly assigned to one of two groups. One group undergoes the experimental treatment initially, while the other group receives the experimental treatment second. After a sufficient period to allow for any treatment effects to diminish (W), the treatments are crossed over, meaning that the group initially receiving the experimental treatment switches to the control treatment, and vice versa. This design allows researchers to assess both the immediate and delayed effects of the treatments on the subjects, providing a comprehensive understanding of the intervention's impact. Multiple cross-over designs may involve several treatments, offering researchers a versatile approach to study the effects of different interventions in a controlled and systematic manner.

Scenario: Investigating the Effect of Different Work Shifts on Nurse Fatigue
In this study, researchers are interested in examining the impact of different work shifts on nurse fatigue. They decide to use a cross-over design to expose nurses to both day and night shifts.

Group Assignment:
Group 1:
 – Initially assigned to work day shifts for a specific period.
 – Later, switched to work night shifts for an equivalent period.
Group 2:
 – Initially assigned to work night shifts for a specific period.
 – Later, switched to work day shifts for an equivalent period.

Intervention:
 – Exposure to different work shifts (day and night) constitutes the intervention.

Washout Period:
A sufficient time period is allowed between the switch of shifts to ensure that any fatigue effects from the previous shift are minimized (washout period, *W*).

Measurement:
Fatigue levels are measured before, during, and after each shift.

Post-study Analysis:
Researchers analyze and compare fatigue levels during day and night shifts within each group.
By utilizing the cross-over design, the study aims to account for individual differences and isolate the impact of different work shifts on nurse fatigue, providing valuable insights for optimizing work schedules and mitigating fatigue-related issues among nursing staff.

2.2.2.2 Quasi-Experimental

Quasi-experimental designs, akin to true-experimental designs, explore cause-and-effect relationships among independent and dependent variables. However, these designs lack one characteristic of true-experimental designs, usually the random assignment of subjects to groups [9]. While quasi-experimental designs prove valuable for assessing intervention effectiveness and are considered closer to natural settings, they are more susceptible to threats to internal and external validity. This heightened susceptibility may impact the confidence and generalizability of the study's findings. The most commonly used quasi-experimental designs include the non-equivalent group pretest–posttest group design, control group interrupted time-series design, single-group interrupted time-series design, and counterbalanced design.

The *non-equivalent pretest–posttest* control group design closely resembles the pretest–posttest control group design, with the key distinction being that subjects are not randomly assigned (NR) to groups. In this design, both groups undergo pretesting (O) and posttesting (O). However, the experimental group alone is subjected to a treatment (X). This design allows researchers to evaluate the impact of the treatment on the experimental group while considering potential initial differences between the groups due to non-random assignment.

Scenario: Assessing the Impact of a Training Program on Nurse Communication Skills
In this study, researchers are interested in evaluating the effectiveness of a communication skills training program for nurses. Due to logistical constraints, random assignment to groups is not feasible, leading to the adoption of a Non-equivalent Pretest–Posttest Control Group Design.

Group Assignment:
Experimental Group (Communication Skills Training):
  Nurses voluntarily opt to participate in the communication skills training program.
  No random assignment is conducted due to practical constraints.
Control Group (Standard Training):
  Nurses who do not participate in the communication skills training.
  Matched with the experimental group based on similar job roles and experience.

Pretesting (O1):
Both groups are assessed on their communication skills before the intervention.

Intervention (X):
The experimental group undergoes the communication skills training program.

Posttesting (O2):
Both groups are reassessed on their communication skills after the completion of the study period.

Analysis:
Researchers compare the change in communication skills between the experimental and control groups.
By employing the Non-equivalent Pretest–Posttest Control Group Design, the study aims to explore whether the communication skills training program has a significant impact on nurses' abilities compared to those who receive standard training. The design acknowledges the lack of random assignment but seeks to control for confounding variables by selecting a control group with similar characteristics.

In the *control group* interrupted time-series design, groups undergo repeated measurements or testing on the same variable over time, with no random assignment (NR) to groups. At some point in the series, the experimental group is exposed to a treatment (X), while the control group remains unexposed to the treatment. This design enables researchers to assess the impact of the treatment by comparing changes over time between the experimental and control groups. The absence of random assignment introduces potential confounding factors, requiring careful consideration of alternative explanations for observed effects.

Scenario: Evaluating the Impact of a New Patient Care Protocol

In this study, researchers aim to assess the effectiveness of a new patient care protocol implemented in a hospital setting. Due to practical considerations, random assignment to groups is not possible, leading to the adoption of a Control Group Interrupted Time Series Design.

Group Assignment:

Experimental Group (New Patient Care Protocol):

> A specific unit or department in the hospital where the new protocol is introduced.
> The introduction is not randomly assigned but is based on the decision of hospital administrators.

Control Group (Standard Patient Care Protocol):

> Another unit or department in the same hospital that continues with the standard patient care protocol.
> Matched with the experimental group based on similar patient demographics, size, and characteristics.

Repeated Measurements Over Time (O1, O2, O3, …):

Both groups are measured or tested repeatedly on relevant variables over an extended period before the introduction of the new patient care protocol.

Intervention (X):

The experimental group receives the new patient care protocol.

Post-Intervention Measurements Over Time (O4, O5, O6, …):

Both groups continue to be measured or tested repeatedly after the introduction of the new patient care protocol.

Analysis:

Researchers compare the trends in outcomes over time between the experimental and control groups.

By using the Control Group Interrupted Time Series Design, the study aims to evaluate the impact of the new patient care protocol while accounting for the natural progression of outcomes over time in both groups. The design acknowledges the absence of random assignment and seeks to control for external factors that may influence the outcomes.

In the *single-group* interrupted time-series design, the researcher conducts repeated measurements on only one group, both before and after exposure to a treatment (X). This design allows for the examination of changes within the same group over time, offering insights into the potential effects of the treatment. However, the absence of a control group limits the ability to attribute observed changes solely to the treatment, as alternative explanations or external factors may contribute to the observed outcomes.

Scenario: Assessing the Impact of a New Nursing Training Program

In this study, researchers aim to assess the impact of a new nursing training program on patient care outcomes. Due to practical constraints, a randomized control group is not feasible, leading to the adoption of a Single-Group Interrupted Time-Series Design.

Group Assignment:

Single Group (Nursing Training Program):

> The entire nursing staff in a specific department or unit of a hospital is considered as a single group.

The nursing training program is implemented for all staff members.

Repeated Measurements Over Time (O1, O2, O3, …):

Patient care outcomes, such as medication administration accuracy or patient satisfaction scores, are measured or tested repeatedly over an extended period before the initiation of the nursing training program.

Intervention (X):

The nursing training program is introduced to enhance the skills and knowledge of the nursing staff.

Post-Intervention Measurements Over Time (O4, O5, O6, …):

Patient care outcomes continue to be measured or tested repeatedly after the implementation of the nursing training program.

Analysis:

Researchers analyze the trends in patient care outcomes over time, focusing on changes that coincide with the introduction of the nursing training program.

By using the Single-Group Interrupted Time-Series Design, the study aims to evaluate the impact of the nursing training program within the same group over time. While acknowledging the absence of a control group, the design allows researchers to observe changes in outcomes before and after the intervention, providing insights into the potential effectiveness of the training program.

The *counterbalanced design* closely resembles the cross-over experimental design, but with the distinction that subjects are not randomly assigned (NR) to different groups. Instead, all groups are exposed to all treatments. One of the most common forms of a counterbalanced design

is the Latin square, where four distinct treatments are administered to four naturally assembled groups or individuals. Following each treatment, each group or individual is posttested. It is crucial to note that the number of treatments and groups must be equal in the Latin square design, as illustrated below.

Scenario: Evaluating the Impact of Different Nursing Shift Schedules

In this study, researchers seek to evaluate the impact of different nursing shift schedules on nurse performance and well-being. Due to logistical challenges and ethical considerations, a randomized control group assignment is not feasible. Instead, a counterbalanced design is employed to assess multiple shift schedules within the same group of nurses.

Participants:

The study involves a group of nurses working in a specific unit or department of a hospital.

Shift Schedules (Treatments):

Four different shift schedules are considered: Day Shift, Evening Shift, Night Shift, and Rotating Shifts.

Each nurse experiences all four shift schedules during the study period.

Posttests After Each Treatment (O1, O2, O3, O4):

Performance metrics, such as medication administration accuracy, patient satisfaction, and nurse well-being, are measured after each period of exposure to a specific shift schedule.

Washout Periods (W):

Between each shift schedule, there is a washout period to allow any potential effects of the previous schedule to diminish.

Randomization within the Group:
While the order of shift schedules is predetermined for each nurse, the counterbalanced design involves randomizing the
order across the group to control for
order effects.

Analysis:
Researchers analyze the data to identify
patterns and differences in nurse performance and well-being associated with
different shift schedules.
By using the Counterbalanced Design, the
study aims to overcome the challenges
of random assignment and provide valuable insights into the impact of various
nursing shift schedules on both objective performance measures and subjective well-being within the same group of
nurses.

The choice of a research design is influenced
by the research question or hypothesis and the
nature of the phenomena under investigation. A
true-experimental design is considered the most
robust in establishing causal effects and internal
validity, which involves controlling factors within
the study that could influence outcomes apart
from the experimental intervention or treatment.
On the other hand, a non-experimental design is
generally considered less strong in terms of internal validity, particularly when assessing cause-
and-effect relationships. However, this does not
imply overall weakness in non-experimental
designs. Their weakness is specifically related to
evaluating cause-and-effect relationships and
establishing internal validity. Interestingly, even
the simplest form of non-experiment, a one-time
survey design involving a single observation (O),
is among the most common research approaches.
For certain research questions, especially those
of a descriptive nature, this design is evidently
strong and highly suitable.

2.3 Sampling

Sampling serves as a crucial foundation for
research endeavors, offering a strategic means to
derive meaningful insights from manageable
subsets of data [10]. The fundamental objective is
to obtain a representative subset, comprising a
limited number of units or cases drawn from a
considerably larger population. This targeted
selection process is pivotal for researchers aiming to draw meaningful insights and make generalizations about the entire population based on
the observed patterns within the sample.
Emphasis is placed on employing precise techniques that result in highly representative samples, closely mirroring the overall population.

Probability sampling, a method rooted in
mathematical probability theories, is commonly
favored by quantitative researchers for its systematic approach to sample selection. The utilization of these techniques ensures a rigorous and
unbiased representation, facilitating robust analyses and valid extrapolations to the larger
population.

The *sample population*, comprising specific
individuals, elements, or cases carefully chosen
from a larger population for a research study, is a
crucial element in this process. Representativeness
is a key consideration, ensuring that the chosen
sample accurately mirrors the diversity and
essential features of the larger population.

Researchers also employ sample *representative sampling*, a methodological approach
focused on selecting samples that faithfully
reflect the characteristics of the entire population.
The goal is to minimize bias and enhance the
validity of research findings by ensuring that the
sample is a balanced and accurate representation
of the broader group. This involves employing
rigorous techniques, often rooted in probability
sampling methods, to systematically and randomly select elements for inclusion in the sample. By prioritizing representativeness,
researchers increase the likelihood of drawing
accurate conclusions and making generalizations

that are applicable beyond the confines of the sampled subset, contributing to the overall robustness and reliability of the research study.

2.3.1 Types of Samples

Researchers in quantitative studies commonly rely on probability sampling, a sampling method grounded in mathematical probability theories. This approach, known as probability sampling, is guided by mathematical principles and probability theories to ensure a systematic and objective selection of elements from a larger population. It stands in contrast to nonprobability sampling techniques, forming a key distinction in approaches to sampling in research methodologies (Fig. 2.2).

Probability sampling techniques are favored by quantitative researchers for their methodical nature and ability to provide statistically valid representations of a population. These methods encompass various strategies such as simple random sampling, stratified sampling, and cluster sampling, each contributing to the overall precision and reliability of the study's findings.

In the broader landscape of sampling methodologies, the dichotomy between probability and nonprobability sampling underscores the importance of adopting rigorous and systematic approaches in quantitative research. Probability sampling not only adheres to mathematical principles but also enhances the generalizability of study results, allowing researchers to make accurate inferences about the larger population based on the characteristics of the selected sample. The utilization of probability sampling approaches reflects a commitment to scientific rigor and statistical validity in quantitative research endeavors.

2.3.1.1 Nonprobability Sampling
Nonprobability sampling is a method of selecting units from a population without assigning a specific probability to each unit is inclusion. Unlike probability sampling, which relies on random

Fig. 2.2 Type of sampling

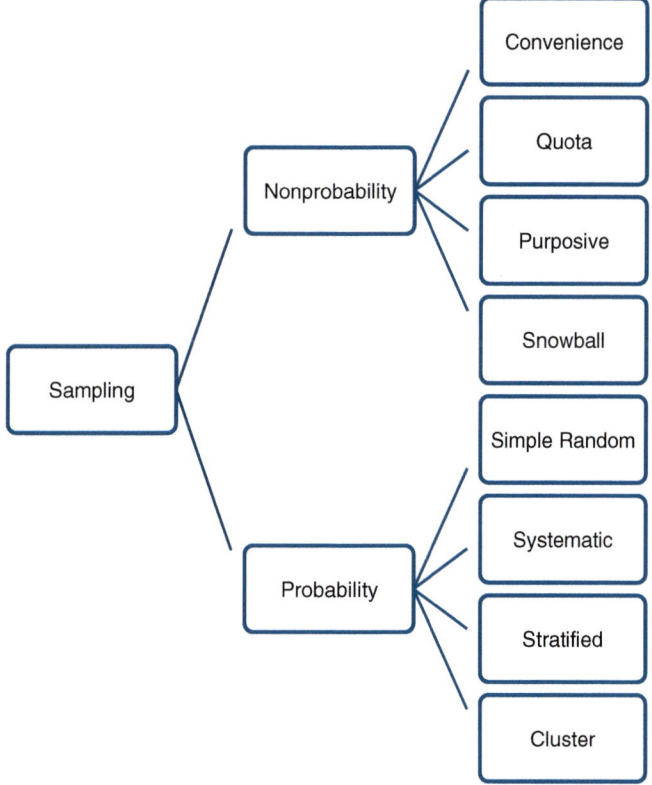

selection, nonprobability sampling does not adhere to a mathematically random approach in choosing units. Consequently, the samples obtained through nonrandom methods often lack representativeness, hindering the generalizability of findings to the broader population. This limitation arises from the absence of a systematic, chance-based selection process, leading to potential biases in the sample composition. In essence, nonprobability sampling methods, such as convenience sampling or purposive sampling, introduce a degree of subjectivity and non-randomness that can impact the validity of research outcomes.

The sample population refers to the group under consideration in a research study, consisting of individuals or elements with shared characteristics. In the context of sampling, it is essential to understand the concept of sample representativeness. A representative sample is one that accurately reflects the key characteristics of the entire population, allowing researchers to make inferences and generalizations with confidence. Achieving sample representativeness involves employing sampling methods that minimize bias and ensure that every subgroup within the population has a fair chance of being included in the sample. This enhances the external validity of the study, enabling researchers to apply their findings to a broader context beyond the sampled group. Consequently, the careful selection of sampling techniques plays a crucial role in determining the extent to which research outcomes can be generalized to the larger population.

Convenience Sampling

Convenience sampling involves the researcher selecting cases for inclusion in the sample based on any convenient criterion. However, the utilization of haphazard sampling, characterized by arbitrary case selection, can yield samples that are effective yet highly unrepresentative of the population, making it an unadvised approach. When cases are chosen haphazardly for their convenience, the resulting sample may significantly distort the true characteristics of the entire population. Despite being cost-effective and quick, the inherent risk of systematic errors associated with

haphazard sampling makes it a less preferable option, with potential consequences more detrimental than having no sample at all. It is crucial for researchers to recognize the limitations of convenience sampling and exercise caution in its application to ensure the reliability and validity of study outcomes.

For example, a researcher is investigating stress levels among nurses working in a busy hospital environment. Due to constraints such as limited time and resources, the researcher opts for convenience sampling by distributing stress questionnaires during a hospital-wide staff meeting. This method allows for quick data collection from nurses who are present at that particular gathering.

However, this convenience sampling approach may introduce bias, as it primarily captures the perspectives of nurses available during the staff meeting. Nurses with varying work shifts, those on leave, or those unable to attend the meeting may be excluded from the study. Consequently, the stress levels reported by the convenience sample might not fully represent the broader spectrum of stress experienced by the entire nursing staff. The findings may be limited in their applicability and may not accurately reflect the diverse stressors faced by nurses across different work settings and schedules.

Quota Sampling

Represents an enhancement compared to convenience sampling. In quota sampling, the researcher initially identifies pertinent population strata and establishes the required number of participants from each stratum. Utilizing information about population characteristics enables researchers to guarantee the representation of diverse segments in the sample, ideally mirroring their proportions in the overall population. Consequently, the sample composition is predetermined with fixed quotas for each category.

For example, in a study focused on understanding patient experiences in a hospital setting, quota sampling can be employed to ensure a comprehensive and representative sample. The researcher identifies key demographic factors such as age and medical condition severity as crucial strata for the study. Two age strata are established: "Under 65 years" and "65 years and above," along with two severity strata: "Mild to Moderate" and "Severe."

To systematically include diverse perspectives, the researcher sets specific quotas for each stratum. For instance, the plan might involve 50 participants from each age group and 30 participants from each severity group. These quotas are determined based on the demographic distribution observed within the hospital's patient population.

The essence of quota sampling lies in its commitment to ensuring proportional representation. By aligning the quotas with the observed proportions in the hospital, the researcher aims to capture the diversity present in the patient population. This structured approach not only facilitates the inclusion of participants from various demographic categories but also guarantees a fixed number of participants from each stratum.

In summary, quota sampling in nursing research provides a methodical and intentional strategy for participant selection, contributing to a more balanced and representative sample. This approach enhances the reliability and validity of the study by capturing a nuanced understanding of patient experiences across different age and severity categories.

Purposive Sampling

Purposive sampling, also known as judgmental sampling, is a strategic research method where researchers intentionally select sample members based on their understanding of the population. In this approach, individuals perceived as representative or possessing significant expertise on the studied issues are deliberately chosen, despite the absence of an external, objective measure to evaluate representativeness. This subjective sampling method proves advantageous in specific contexts, particularly when dealing with populations presenting challenges in accessibility or measurement.

This valid and tailored approach is often employed in unique circumstances, leveraging the expertise of knowledgeable individuals to select cases or address specific research objectives. Purposive sampling is particularly valuable when faced with populations that pose challenges in terms of accessibility or measurement, as the researcher seeks a targeted and intentional representation of specific characteristics within the population. This intentional selection process facilitates a more focused and insightful study.

Referred to as judgmental or selective sampling, purposeful sampling involves the conscious selection of certain participants, elements, events, or incidents for inclusion in the study. The flexibility of purposive sampling allows researchers to tailor their approach based on the unique demands of the study, making it a valuable tool in the researcher's toolkit for gathering nuanced insights in diverse research contexts. In a concrete example, a research project focusing on exploring the experiences of nurses managing palliative care patients employs purposive sampling by intentionally selecting participants with extensive experience in palliative care nursing. This ensures a sample with rich insights into the specific challenges and coping strategies in this field, contributing to a more comprehensive understanding of the subject matter.

Snowball Sampling

Snowball sampling, also known as network, chain referral, or reputational sampling, is a strategic method for identifying and sampling cases within a network. It initiates with one or a few individuals or cases and then expands based on connections to the initial cases. Participants are chosen based on specific research criteria, and subsequently, these respondents are prompted to suggest other individuals who align with the target population, ultimately becoming subjects in the sample. This ongoing process results in a continual growth of the sample size. This sampling approach is particularly effective in situations where the targeted population is a minority or where the identification of specific subjects is challenging due to various factors.

Moreover, snowball sampling proves beneficial when aiming to reach populations that are hard to access, ensuring a more comprehensive representation in the study. By capitalizing on existing connections and referrals, this method becomes especially valuable in situations where traditional sampling techniques might be impractical or insufficient for capturing the diversity within a particular population. The iterative nature of snowball sampling allows for the inclusion of individuals who might otherwise be overlooked in more conventional sampling approaches.

For example, in a nursing study exploring the challenges faced by caregivers of pediatric cancer patients, the researcher begins by conducting interviews with a few caregivers identified through a support group. Subsequently, these initial participants refer the researcher to others in similar situations, creating a snowball effect in participant recruitment.

2.3.1.2 Probability Sampling

Probability sampling is a method where each unit in a population has a specifiable chance of being selected, meaning that all individuals in the population have an equal chance of being chosen. The rationale for employing this technique is to produce a sample that accurately mirrors the characteristics of the overall population. It is important to note that while random sampling does not ensure that every sample precisely represents the population, it does mean that the majority of random samples will closely approximate the population most of the time. Additionally, the probability of a specific sample being accurate can be calculated.

In probability sampling, each unit within a population has an identifiable likelihood of being chosen, ensuring that all individuals in the population have an equal chance of being selected. The aim is to create a sample that is representative of the broader population. It is essential to recognize that while random sampling doesn't guarantee perfect representation in every instance, it does indicate that the majority of random samples will closely align with the population characteristics most of the time. Furthermore, this approach allows for the calculation of the probability associated with the accuracy of a particular sample.

2.3.1.3 Simple Random Sampling

Simple random sampling, the most fundamental of probability sampling plans, involves the random selection of elements from a sampling frame. This basic strategy in probability sampling allows researchers to employ various methods for random selection, with the approach being limited only by the researcher's imagination. In instances where the sampling frame is small, researchers can creatively use slips of paper with names, placing them into a container, thoroughly mixing them, and then drawing them out one at a time until the desired sample size is reached. Another commonly utilized method for random selection is through the use of a computer program, providing efficiency and widespread applicability in selecting study participants.

Randomization techniques, such as drawing numbers from a hat or container, using a table of random numbers, employing a coin toss, the sealed opaque envelope technique, or a computer program, can be employed for selecting random samples. Simple random sampling is particularly fitting when the characteristics of all population units are similar, indicating homogeneity.

However, in the case of a population with diverse characteristics, i.e., heterogeneity, relying solely on simple random sampling might be imprudent when aiming to obtain a representative sample that captures the main variables being studied.

For example, in a study investigating the types of hand hygiene practices among nurses in a hospital, a researcher employs simple random sampling to categorize the nursing staff into two groups: Group one, practicing hand sanitizer usage, and Group two, relying on traditional hand washing. Each nurse in the hospital is assigned a unique identification number through computer randomization techniques. The researcher then randomly selects a representative sample from this pool, ensuring an unbiased representation of nurses from both groups. This approach allows the findings to shed light on the prevalence and effectiveness of hand hygiene practices in the broader nursing population within the hospital.

Systematic Sampling

Systematic sampling emerges as another viable probability sampling strategy, particularly applicable in situations where the population exhibits heterogeneity. This approach often entails selecting every nth number, representing any randomly chosen number, from a sequentially numbered list of all units in the population. The selection of every nth number ensures a consistent interval between the listed numbers. For this strategy to be effective, the researcher must ensure that the population units are randomly listed, the nth number is chosen randomly before selecting the first population unit for the sample, and the initial unit is selected through a random process. For instance, with a population size (N) of 1000 and a desired sample size (n) of 100, the calculated k is 10. Consequently, the researcher would include every tenth person on the list in the sample.

In a study aimed at assessing medication administration practices in a large hospital with a diverse nursing staff, the researcher has an ordered list of all registered nurses working in different units of the hospital, totalling 700 nurses. If the researcher aims for a sample size (n) of 100 nurses, and the total population size (N) is 700, the calculated k (the interval between selections) would be 700/100 = 7. Therefore, the researcher would include every seventh nurse from the ordered list of registered nurses in the sample.

Stratified Sampling

In stratified random sampling, the initial step involves the division of the population into subpopulations, known as strata, based on additional information that defines a characteristic of the population. For instance, these strata could be delineated by gender, age, education, experience, or illness condition. Subsequently, the researcher randomly selects samples from each of these subpopulations. Generally, stratified sampling is deemed more representative of the overall population compared to simple random sampling, particularly when the stratum information is accurate.

For example, in a nursing study assessing the impact of a new intervention on stress reduction among hospital nurses, the researcher employs stratified random sampling based on years of experience. The nursing staff is divided into three strata: less than 5 years, 5–15 years, and more than 15 years. By randomly selecting nurses from each stratum, the study ensures representation across different experience levels, enhancing the ability to draw nuanced conclusions about the intervention's effectiveness within the diverse nursing staff.

Cluster Sampling

In the context of cluster sampling, a cluster is defined as a "group of similar things." Occasionally, the units of the study population naturally form clusters. This method involves dividing the population into clusters, with elements from each cluster chosen as subjects for the study. Each cluster contains similar types of data, resulting in heterogeneous data within the cluster and homogeneous data across clusters. Consequently, the researcher can choose one or more clusters to collect the data.

Using area clusters as an example, consider a research study focused on implementing a protocol to reduce medication errors among nurses. The study's objectives include gathering feedback, assessing adherence to the protocol, and identifying challenges or successes. The sampling involves nurses from various hospital departments, such as the emergency department, intensive care unit, medical-surgical unit, and pediatrics unit. Through cluster sampling, the researcher randomly selects a subset of departments from the complete list of hospital departments. For instance, they might randomly choose the emergency department, intensive care unit, and pediatrics unit. This approach ensures a representative sample from diverse hospital departments, providing a comprehensive understanding of how the new protocol is implemented across different areas of patient care. However, it is essential to note that while cluster sampling is cost-efficient, it may lack generalizability.

2.4   Data Collection

Data collection is the precise and systematic gathering of information relevant to the research purpose or the specific objectives, questions, or hypotheses of a study. It involves the deliberate and organized collection of data points or facts from various sources, which can include surveys, experiments, interviews, observations, or existing records. The goal of data collection is to compile a comprehensive and accurate set of information that serves as the foundation for subsequent analysis, interpretation, and decision-making. Effective data collection is crucial for ensuring the reliability and validity of research findings, enabling researchers to draw meaningful conclusions and insights based on the gathered information.

After identifying the data requirements, the subsequent step involves selecting an appropriate data collection method for each variable. When reviewing data needs, researchers should determine the most effective way to capture each variable based on its conceptual or theoretical definition. Research considerations are not the sole factors guiding decisions about data collection methods; ethical considerations, budget constraints, the availability of qualified staff for data collection, time constraints, and the anticipated impact on participants and other stakeholders, such as hospital staff or participants' families, also play a crucial role. Data collection is typically the most costly and time-consuming aspect of a study. Consequently, researchers often have to make compromises regarding the type or quantity of data collected.

Quantitative research revolves around the methodical gathering and analysis of numerical data, serving as the cornerstone for informed decision-making and conclusive insights. The data collection process in quantitative nursing studies plays a pivotal role, establishing the foundation for robust analysis and meaningful interpretation. Decisions regarding research design often operate independently of the chosen data collection methods in nursing studies. The main data collection methods—self-reports, observa-

tion, and biophysiologic measures—can involve either existing data or original data created specifically for research. The specific choice of a data collection method may be influenced by the research question, guiding its placement along the four continua described earlier.

2.4.1   Self-Reporting

Self-reports serve as a valuable method for acquiring information by directly questioning individuals, a process integral to data collection in various fields, particularly in nursing studies. For instance, if our focus is on exploring nursing staff's perspectives on interprofessional collaboration, job-related stressors, or adherence to infection control protocols, engaging in discussions and querying individuals emerges as a primary methodology. The distinctive ability of humans to communicate verbally at an advanced level underscores the significance of direct questioning in the toolkit of nurse researchers for data collection.

The majority of nursing studies heavily rely on data collected through self-reports, emphasizing the method's strength in terms of directness and versatility. When seeking insights into people's thoughts, emotions, or beliefs, the most efficient strategy involves directly asking them. A persuasive rationale in favor of the self-report method is its often-demonstrated effectiveness in eliciting information that might be difficult or even impossible to gather using alternative approaches. While certain behaviors can be publicly observed, confidential actions like instances of school bullying, student engagement in academic dishonesty, or sensitive mental health concerns are usually outside the purview of direct observation by researchers. Moreover, observers can only witness behaviors occurring during the study, limiting the scope of observation. Self-reports, on the other hand, enable researchers to gather retrospective data about past activities or obtain projections regarding future behaviors.

Although observations can sometimes offer insights into feelings, values, opinions, and motives, there is an inherent challenge in ensuring an exact correspondence between observed behaviors and genuine emotions. People's actions may not always accurately reflect their state of mind. In such instances, self-report methods prove valuable in capturing psychological characteristics through direct communication with participants, offering a nuanced understanding that goes beyond mere behavioral observation.

While verbal reporting methods offer advantages, they also entail certain limitations. The primary concern revolves around questioning the credibility and precision of self-reports: How can we reliably ascertain the authenticity of respondents' expressed feelings or actions? The challenge intensifies when respondents may be hesitant to disclose truthful information, particularly if it involves illegal or socially unacceptable behavior. Investigators often find themselves in a predicament, compelled to assume the honesty of respondents due to a lack of alternative methods.

Yet, the inherent human tendency to portray oneself positively introduces a potential conflict with the truth. Individuals may be inclined to present a more favorable version of their feelings or actions. This inclination to project a positive image raises questions about the reliability of the data collected through self-reports. Therefore, researchers engaged in gathering self-report data need to explicitly recognize the method's inherent limitations. They should be prepared to navigate these complexities when interpreting results, ensuring a nuanced understanding that accounts for potential biases introduced by the respondents' desire to present themselves in a positive light.

2.4.2 Observation

Observation serves as a valuable alternative to self-reports in tackling specific research challenges, allowing researchers to directly observe people's behavior. Nurse researchers often rely on this method to acquire information essential for demonstrating nursing effectiveness and identifying clues to enhance nursing practices. The intrinsic appeal of observation lies in its ability to directly capture a record of behaviors and events. Moreover, with an observational approach, the observers themselves—human professionals—are utilized as measuring instruments, providing a uniquely sensitive and intelligent tool. This distinctive quality reinforces the effectiveness of observational research in the nuanced and dynamic field of nursing.

Observations can take place in controlled laboratory environments or in natural, real-world settings. Furthermore, the process of observation can occur either directly through human senses or with the assistance of technical tools such as video equipment and tape recorders. This versatility makes observation a dynamic and adaptable method of collecting data. Similar to self-report techniques, observational methods can exhibit varying degrees of structure. For instance, a researcher might choose to observe nurses' interactions with patients in an unstructured manner, capturing detailed narrative notes about the nuanced use of touch. Alternatively, the researcher could opt for a more structured approach by tallying the frequency of specific types of touching employed by nurses, following a predetermined classification system. This flexibility allows researchers to tailor their observational methods to the specific nuances of the research question at hand.

Observational methods present a versatile toolkit for gathering a diverse range of information, extending beyond general characteristics to specific instances like hand hygiene compliance in intensive care units (ICUs). By directly observing healthcare professionals, researchers can gain insights into adherence to hand hygiene protocols, a critical aspect of patient care. In the context of hand hygiene compliance in ICUs, observational methods become instrumental. Researchers can meticulously observe healthcare practitioners during routine activities, noting instances of hand hygiene practices. This includes both verbal aspects, such as communication during patient care, and nonverbal cues like facial expressions, which may reflect the conscientiousness of following hygiene protocols. Furthermore, observational methods allow for the documentation of various activities related to hand hygiene within ICUs, offering a comprehensive understanding. This might involve observing the frequency and techniques of handwashing or the utilization of hand sanitizers. Additionally, this approach provides a direct and nuanced perspective, allowing researchers to uncover critical insights into healthcare practices for the betterment of patient safety and overall quality of care.

In a nursing research laboratory, professionals might undertake an observational study to explore the efficacy of a newly implemented patient care protocol. Nurses could be observed as they interact with simulated patients or use advanced medical equipment. This laboratory setting allows researchers to closely monitor and document how nurses adhere to the prescribed procedures, ensuring precision and consistency in the application of the new protocol. For instance, researchers may observe the nurses' use of personal protective equipment, their communication with the simulated patients, and their overall adherence to infection control measures. The controlled laboratory environment provides a controlled and standardized setting, enabling researchers to pinpoint specific behaviors and outcomes related to the implemented protocol. Observing nursing practices in a laboratory setting allows for meticulous data collection, providing valuable insights into the practical application of protocols. The findings from such observations can contribute to refining and optimizing nursing practices for enhanced patient care outcomes.

The observational approach, while highly valuable, comes with its set of challenges. These challenges encompass potential ethical dilemmas, the risk of altered behavior from the person being observed when the observer is conspicuous, and a significant rate of refusal to cooperate. Additionally, a pervasive issue lies in the susceptibility of observational data to observer biases. Objective observations often encounter interference from various factors. The emotions, prejudices, attitudes, and values of observers can lead to faulty inferences, potentially compromising the accuracy of the findings. Personal interests and commitments might influence what observers perceive, directing their attention toward what they wish to see rather than maintaining impartiality. Furthermore, the anticipation of what is expected to be observed can impact the actual observations, potentially introducing bias into the collected data. Hasty decisions made before acquiring sufficient information may result in erroneous classifications or premature conclusions.

Although it proves challenging to completely eliminate observational biases, their impact can be mitigated through meticulous training. By equipping observers with the necessary tools and skills to navigate these challenges, researchers can enhance the reliability and validity of observational data. This approach ensures a more accurate representation of the behaviors and events under study, reinforcing the credibility of findings derived from the observational method.

2.4.3   Biophysiologic Measures

In the realm of nursing research, there has been a notable shift toward heightened clinical, patient-centric investigations. This shift has led to an increased reliance on measures assessing the physiological status of subjects, often employing quantitative biophysiologic measures. Typically requiring specialized technical instruments and equipment as well as specific training for result interpretation, these measures focus on physiological and physical variables.

Physiological measurements are essential tools in understanding and monitoring the functions of living organisms. These measurements can be broadly classified into two primary categories: in vivo and in vitro. In vivo measurements involve the direct assessment of physiological parameters within or on a living organism. This approach provides real-time data, offering insights into the dynamic functioning of biological systems. Examples of in vivo measurements include monitoring oxygen saturation levels, measuring blood pressure, and recording body temperature in humans.

In contrast, in vitro measurements are conducted outside the organism's body, typically in controlled laboratory settings. This approach allows researchers to analyze biological components or processes in isolation, providing a more controlled and detailed examination. An example of in vitro measurement is determining the concentration of serum potassium in a blood sample or Hemo Glucose Test (HGT).

Researchers often utilize a combination of in vivo and in vitro measurements to obtain a comprehensive understanding of physiological processes. This dual approach allows for a more nuanced exploration of biological functions, providing valuable insights into health, disease, and the effects of interventions. Whether monitoring vital signs in a patient or conducting experiments in a laboratory, the choice between in vivo and in vitro measurements depends on the research objectives and the level of control required over experimental conditions.

Healthcare settings, where nurses operate, are frequently equipped with a diverse array of technical instruments designed for measuring physiological functions. While the equipment for obtaining physiologic measurements tends to be costly, its widespread availability in healthcare settings can minimize or eliminate costs for nurse researchers. For example, a nurse researcher is investigating respiratory health. In this case, the nurse could employ pulse oximeters to measure oxygen saturation levels in patients. If two nurses use the same type of pulse oximeter on a patient, they should obtain identical oxygen saturation readings. This uniformity in measurements across different nurses and equipment highlights the objectivity and consistency of biophysiologic measures.

Furthermore, the reliability extends to scenarios involving blood pressure monitoring. Consider two nurses utilizing automated blood pressure cuffs on the same patient. Assuming proper calibration and functionality, both nurses should record matching blood pressure readings, reinforcing the dependability of biophysiologic measures in providing consistent and objective data. This demonstrates the robustness of biophysiologic measures in capturing accurate and

reliable information, ensuring that healthcare professionals can trust the objectivity of their measurements in various clinical contexts.

Despite their advantages, physiologic measurements come with certain drawbacks. The technical nature of the equipment may lead non-engineers to underestimate its limitations, fostering unwarranted faith in its accuracy. Nevertheless, biophysiologic measures consistently yield data of exceptionally high quality due to their relative precision and sensitivity, setting them apart from measures of psychological phenomena like self-report assessments of anxiety or pain.

2.5   Data Analysis

Data analysis is a multifaceted process encompassing the meticulous examination, purification, transformation, and modeling of data to extract crucial insights. Its primary purpose is to facilitate decision-making by uncovering significant information and proposing well-founded conclusions. In this context, quantitative data analysis emerges as a powerful approach, relying on numerical scores or ratings to provide tangible and easily calculable results. This method proves invaluable in evaluation processes, offering quantifiable outcomes that are not only efficient but also conducive to effective presentation. The richness of quantitative assessment data lies in its diverse sources, derived from a myriad of assessment measures.

Statistical analyses encompass techniques used to scrutinize, condense, and derive meaning from the numerical data collected. This categorization of statistics distinguishes between descriptive and inferential statistics. Descriptive statistics serve as summary measures, aiding researchers in organizing data to extract meaning and gain insights. These statistics are computed to depict the characteristics of the sample and the key study variables. In contrast, inferential statistics are crafted to address objectives, questions, and hypotheses in studies, allowing researchers to make informed inferences from the study sample to the broader target population. Inferential analyses are conducted to uncover relationships, test predictions, and discern group differences in studies.

2.5.1 Level of Measurement

Descriptive statistics encompass measures of frequency, central tendency, and variability, while inferential statistics include measures of relations and effects. Scientists have established a categorization system for measures, crucial because the type of analysis possible depends on the measurement level. The four primary levels of measurement are nominal, ordinal, interval, and ratio [11].

2.5.1.1 Nominal
Nominal measurement, falling within the broader realm of measurement, involves the assignment of numbers to categorize characteristics distinctly. These categories must be both exhaustive and mutually exclusive and can also be derived from word data. Variables well-suited for nominal measurement encompass aspects like religious denomination, gender, socioeconomic status, and membership in experimental or control treatment groups. This form of measurement is utilized when data can be organized into categories with defined properties, yet these categories lack a meaningful rank order. For example, researchers might categorize participants by gender, assigning the number 1 to males and 2 to females, but these numbers hold no intrinsic significance; the number 2 does not imply "more than" 1. Reversing the code, using 1 for females and 2 for males, would be equally acceptable. In nominal measurement, the qualitative distinctions between categories persist, but there is no quantitative hierarchy established.

2.5.1.2 Ordinal
Ordinal-level measurement involves the assignment of numbers to represent a rank order, based on the standing of each research participant's score relative to others. Examples include the rank order of scores from low to high and Likert

scale ratings indicating levels of agreement, such as strongly agree, agree, disagree, and strongly disagree. In this measurement type, the numbers assigned reflect the rank order (first, second, third, etc.) of the entities being assessed. For instance, when measuring the intensity of depression, various levels of depression may be identified, categorized as excruciating, severe, moderate, mild, and no depression. However, in ordinal measurement, the intervals between ranked categories are not assumed to be equal. For example, the difference between mild and moderate depression may be greater than that between excruciating and severe depression. As a result, ordinal data are recognized for having unequal intervals.

Numerous scales employed in nursing research often fall under the category of ordinal measurement. One illustrative example is the Nurses Job Satisfaction Scale, designed to rank the levels of job satisfaction among nurses. Through this scale, researchers assess and assign numbers to indicate the ordinal order of nurses' satisfaction levels, allowing for the identification of variations in job satisfaction across different categories. For instance, the scale might categorize satisfaction levels as follows:

1 = Low
2 = Moderate
3 = High
4 = Very high

This categorization enables the ranking of nurses based on their perceived job satisfaction without assuming equal intervals between these ordinal categories. This approach acknowledges qualitative distinctions while recognizing that the intervals between satisfaction levels may not be uniform.

2.5.1.3 Interval
Interval-level measurement involves using scales with equal numerical distances between intervals, characterized by mutually exclusive, exhaustive, and ranked categories, assuming a continuum of values. This enables a more precise

definition of attribute magnitude, with the requirement that intervals between categories are uniform. However, a notable feature is the absence of a true zero point, preventing the provision of an absolute amount for the attribute.

A classic example of an interval scale is temperature, where the differences between degrees are consistent. For instance, the difference between 70 and 80 °F is 10 °F, identical to the difference between 30 and 40 °F. While temperature changes can be precisely measured, a temperature of 0 °F does not indicate the absence of temperature but rather represents a point on the scale.

Another example of an interval scale is the intelligence quotient (IQ) scores. IQ scores are measured on an interval scale, wherein the intervals between scores are considered uniform. For instance, the difference between an IQ score of 100 and 110 is deemed equivalent to the difference between 120 and 130. This allows for a meaningful interpretation of the differences in intelligence levels based on IQ scores. However, it is crucial to recognize that a score of 0 in IQ does not indicate the absence of intelligence but represents a point on the scale.

2.5.1.4 Ratio

Ratio measurement represents the highest level of measurement, characterized by a rational and meaningful zero point. In ratio scales, numerical values not only indicate the rank-ordering of objects based on a critical attribute but also convey information about the intervals between objects and the absolute magnitude of the attribute. This type of measurement is particularly applicable to physical measures where a true zero value is possible. For instance, a person's weight measured on a ratio scale allows for meaningful statements, such as stating that an individual weighing 100 kg is twice as heavy as someone weighing 50 kg. The presence of an absolute zero in ratio scales enables the use of all arithmetic operations, making it permissible to add, subtract, multiply, and divide these numbers. Consequently, statistical procedures suitable for interval-level data are also applicable to ratio level data. Another example of ratio measure-

ment includes vital signs (pulse rate, respiratory rate, and blood pressure) and the Celsius (centigrade) scale of temperature.

2.5.2   Descriptive Statistics

Descriptive statistics, as previously introduced, enable researchers to structure numerical data in a way that provides meaning and enhances understanding. In any research involving numerical data, the initial step in data analysis involves the application of descriptive statistics. In some studies, data analysis is exclusively focused on descriptive statistics, while in contrast, other studies use descriptive statistics primarily to depict the characteristics of the sample and the values derived from measuring dependent or research variables. This section presents various descriptive statistics, such as frequency distributions, percentages, measures of central tendency, measures of dispersion, and standardized scores.

For instance, when examining ordinal data, which involves variables with ordered categories, descriptive statistics can help illustrate the distribution of these categories and provide insights into the order and spread within the data. In an ordinal study, researchers might employ descriptive statistics to present the frequency of responses in each ordered category, offering a clearer understanding of the distribution patterns and tendencies within the dataset.

2.5.2.1 Frequency Distribution

Frequency distributions play a crucial role in the realm of quantitative research as they serve as a systematic method to organize and summarize datasets. At their core, these distributions offer a clear and concise representation of how frequently each value or range of values occurs within the data. The initial step involves organizing raw data, where individual scores are listed alongside the frequency of their occurrence. This organization facilitates a deeper understanding of the distribution's patterns, enabling researchers to discern central tendencies, variability, and potential outliers.

Most studies have some categorical data that are presented in the form of an ungrouped frequency distribution, in which a table is developed to display all numerical values obtained for a particular variable. This approach is generally used on discrete rather than continuous data. Examples of data commonly organized in this manner are gender, ethnicity, marital status, diagnoses of study participants, and values obtained from the measurement of selected research and dependent variables.

Consider the dataset presented in Table 2.1, comprising 50 patients' heart rate measurements (beats per minute) of patients in a hospital. Merely inspecting the raw numbers does not provide a clear understanding of the data. However, through an organized scheme, depicted in Table 2.2, key insights become apparent. This organized presentation allows for a quick grasp of the highest and lowest heart rates, the most common rate, the central clustering of scores, and the total sample size. Table 2.2 example of frequencies, where each score is displayed alongside the number of participants receiving that particular score. This structured approach unveils patterns and characteristics that were not immediately evident in the raw, unorganized data.

In the realm of nursing research, the application of frequency distribution is diverse and impactful. One common use involves the analysis of patient demographics, encompassing factors such as age, gender, and ethnicity. Moreover, in the assessment of clinical measurements, variables such as blood pressure, heart rate, and temperature are subjected to frequency distribution analysis to glean insights into the distribution of values among patients. Furthermore, frequency distributions are instrumental in evaluating the effectiveness of healthcare interventions, allowing researchers to analyze changes in relevant

variables over time and make informed decisions based on the observed patterns.

Table 2.3 is an example of how frequency distributions for demographic variables related to heart rate patients ($N = 50$) might be presented in a study format in a journal. Tables or graphs, such as pie charts, bar charts, and line graphs, are commonly used to present frequency distributions. In Fig. 2.3, visual representations of the age distribution by group from Table 2.3 are depicted. It is worth observing in the bar and line graphs that the data distribution exhibits a normal curve.

2.5.2.2 Central Tendency

A measure of central tendency is a singular value that aims to characterize a dataset by pinpointing its central position [12]. These measures are also referred to as measures of central location and

Table 2.2 Frequency distribution for the heart rates of 50 patients

Heart rate	Frequency	Percent	Cumulative percent
68	4	8	8
72	9	18	26
75	4	8	34
76	4	8	42
78	8	16	58
80	4	8	66
84	4	8	74
85	4	8	82
88	5	10	92
90	4	8	100
Total	50	100	

The "Heart Rate" column represents the individual heart rates in ascending order
The "Frequency" column indicates how many times each heart rate occurs in the dataset
The "Percent" column represents the percentage of each heart rate's frequency relative to the total number of patients (50)
The "Cumulative Percent" column shows the running total of percentages, which reaches 100% at the end

Table 2.1 Result of heart rate of 50 patients

72	90	80	68	88	78	78	76	72	75
78	78	76	72	75	84	85	72	90	80
84	85	72	90	80	68	88	78	78	76
68	88	78	78	76	72	75	84	85	72
72	75	84	85	72	90	80	68	88	88

Table 2.3 Descriptive statistics of demographic variables for heart rate patients ($N = 50$)

Variable	Frequency	Percentage (%)
Gender		
Male	25	50
Female	25	50
Age		
20–30	1	2
30–40	16	32
40–50	17	34
50–60	14	28
60–70	2	4
Marital status		
Married	25	50
Single	15	30
Others	10	20

fall under the category of summary statistics. Essentially, a measure of central tendency is a numerical representation of the typical value within a set of numbers. Three well-known measures in this category are the mean, median, and mode. While the mean, often known as the average, is likely the most familiar, there are others like the median and mode. The mean, median, and mode are all legitimate measures of central tendency, each suitable under different circumstances. The choice of which to use depends on the characteristics of the dataset and specific conditions.

2.5.2.3 Mode

The mode is the numerical value or score that occurs with the greatest frequency; however, it does not necessarily indicate the center of the data set. The mode is particularly suitable as a measure of central tendency for nominal data. In Table 2.2, representing the heart rates of 50 patients, the mode is the score of 5, which appeared nine times in the data set. The mode proves useful in describing the typical study participant or identifying the most frequently occurring value on a scale item (refer to Fig. 2.3). Importantly, a data set can have more than one mode. When two modes exist, the data set is referred to as a bimodal distribution. If there are more than two modes, the data set is described as multimodal.

Median

The median serves as the midpoint or the value at the precise center of an ungrouped frequency distribution, representing the 50th percentile. Calculating the median involves arranging the scores in ascending or descending order. In cases with an odd number of scores, the median is the middle value; for an even number, it is the average of the two middle scores. This means that the median may not necessarily be one of the actual scores in the dataset. Unlike the mean, the median remains unaffected by extreme or outlier scores. It is especially suited for ordinal data, offering a reliable measure of central tendency. In the context of the heart rate data given in Table 2.2, the median is determined to be 78.

A fundamental characteristic of the median is its disregard for the specific quantitative values of scores. Instead, it serves as an indicator of the average position within a distribution and remains impervious to extreme values. For instance, consider the set of numbers:

$$2, 4, 6, 8, 10, 11, 12, 14, 16, 18, 99.$$

The median, determined as 11, represents the middle value when the data is arranged in ascending order. Notably, even with a substantial increase in the last value from 18 to 99, the median remains unchanged at 11.

Mean

The most frequently utilized measure of central tendency is the mean, calculated as the sum of scores divided by the total number of scores. The formula for calculating the mean ($\bar{X}$) is as follows:

$$\bar{X} = \frac{\Sigma X}{N},$$

where:

- $\bar{X}$ is the mean,
- ΣX represents the sum of all individual scores,
- N is the total number of scores in the dataset.

For example, consider the set of numbers: 5, 8, 6, 8, 11, 11, 12, 15, 16, 18.

Fig. 2.3 Common graphic displays for frequency distributions include bar graphs, histograms, and pie charts

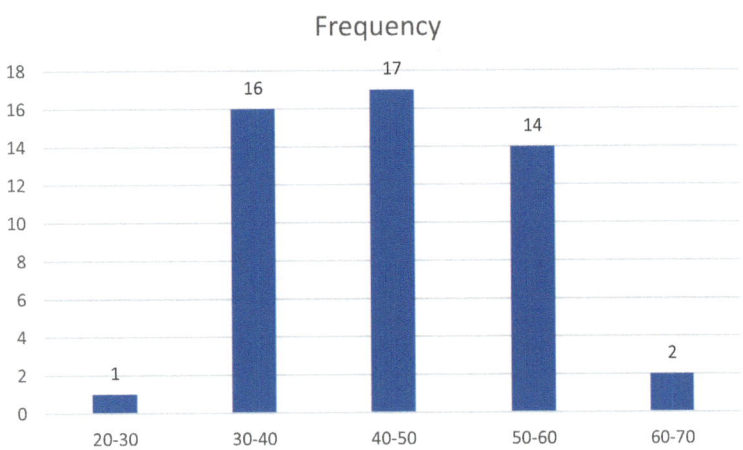

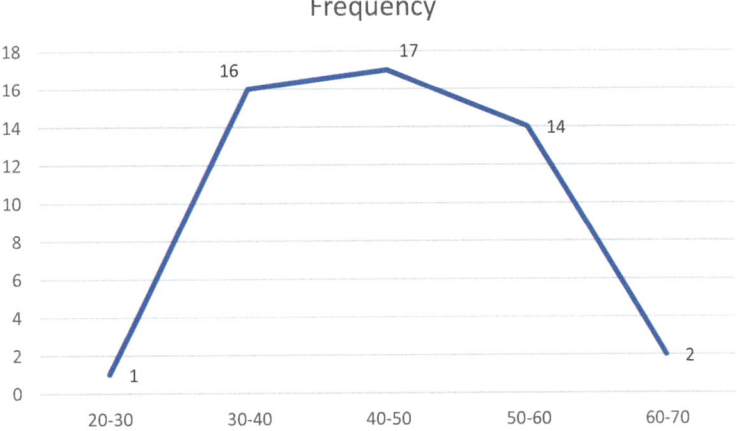

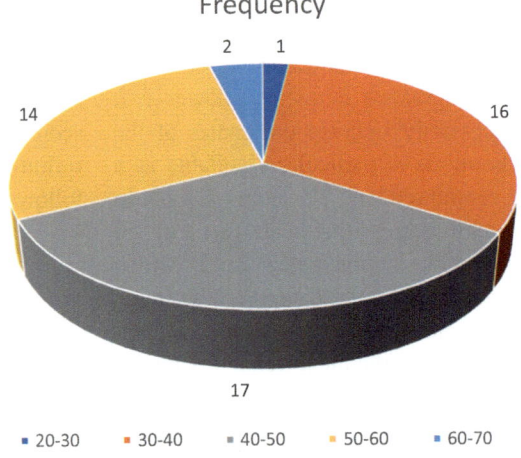

$$\bar{X} = \frac{5+8+6+8+11+11+12+15+16+18}{11} = 10$$

Similar to the median, the mean may not correspond to an actual value within the dataset. The mean is particularly suitable for interval- and ratio level data. However, in studies with outliers, the mean is highly influenced by these extreme values, and the median might be the preferred measure of central tendency reported in the research findings. For instance, in the context of the heart rate data for 50 patients in Table 2.2, the mean is determined to be 78.88.

2.5.2.4 Dispersion

Measures of dispersion also referred to as variability, assess the differences among individual members of a sample. They are aptly named as they reveal how data are spread around the means, offering insights into the distribution of values. Unlike measures of central tendency, these dispersion measures provide information about the extent of individual differences within the data. They convey the degree of variability or deviation among individual scores. When scores are similar, indicating homogeneity, measures of variability are small. Conversely, a heterogeneous sample exhibits a broad range of scores, signifying greater variation among individual data points.

2.5.2.5 Range

The statistical range represents the gap between the highest and lowest values within a dataset. However, due to its dependence on specific samples, it is considered an unreliable measure of variability. Table 2.4 illustrates the recorded heart rate measurements of 10 patients in both the experimental and control groups of a study. Although both groups have a mean of 82 and medians of 81 for the control group and 82 for the experimental group, the datasets differ significantly. The experimental group's heart rates exhibit more diversity, ranging from 65 to 105, with a broader range of 40. In contrast, the control group's heart rates range from 70 to 92, with

Table 2.4 Example of range in heart rate in a study with two groups

	Control	Experimental
	70	65
	75	72
	75	73
	80	76
	80	81
	82	83
	86	87
	88	88
	92	90
	92	105
Median	81	82
Mean	82	82
Range	22	40
Standard deviation	7.47	11.36

a narrower range of 22. When comparing data, a smaller range indicates more consistent data, while a larger range suggests greater variability.

Its sensitivity to outliers makes it less reliable in the presence of extreme values, as a single outlier can disproportionately influence the measure. Additionally, the range does not consider the distribution pattern of values within the dataset; it merely reflects the spread between the two extreme values.

Semi-quartile Range

The semi-interquartile range, often known as the semi-IQR or semi-quartile range, is a measure of statistical dispersion that focuses on the spread of the central half of a dataset. It is calculated as half the difference between the first quartile ($Q1$) and the third quartile ($Q3$). Quartiles divide a dataset into four equal parts, and the semi-interquartile range provides insights into the variability of the middle 50% of the data.

The formula for the semi-interquartile range is

$$\text{Semi IQR} = \frac{Q3 - Q1}{2}$$

Figure 2.4 shows the data of 20 patients' heart rates.

First, find the first quartile ($Q1$) and third quartile ($Q3$).

65	70	72	74	75	76	77	78	79	80	80	82	83	85	86	88	89	90	92	95
			$Q_1 = 75.5$						Median = 80						$Q_3 = 87$				

Fig. 2.4 Example of the semi-quartile range calculation

Fig. 2.5 Example of the percentile calculation

22	24	26	28	30	32	34	36	38	40	42	44
		25th Percentile = 26				Median = 33		75th Percentile = 38			

– $Q1$ is the median of the lower half of the data: $\dfrac{75 + 76}{2} = 75.5$.

– $Q3$ is the median of the upper half of the data: $\dfrac{86 + 88}{2} = 87$.

Calculate the semi-interquartile range:

$$\text{Semi IQR} = \frac{87 - 75.5}{2} = 5.75$$

In this example, the semi-interquartile range is 5.75, providing a measure of the spread of the middle 50% of the exam scores. It is particularly useful in situations where extreme values might disproportionately influence the full interquartile range.

Percentile

A percentile serves as a ranking measure, indicating the percentage of cases in a dataset that a particular value surpasses. Essential percentiles include the median, corresponding to the 50th percentile, the first quartile at the 25th percentile, and the third quartile at the 75th percentile. These percentiles offer valuable insights into the distribution of values within a dataset, helping to identify key positions and understand how specific values compare relative to the entire dataset.

Figure 2.5 illustrates the example of the body mass index (BMI) of 12 patients, illustrating the calculation of percentiles as follows:

- Calculate the Median (50th Percentile):

$$\text{Median} = \frac{32 + 34}{2} = 33$$

- Calculate the First Quartile (25th Percentile):
  - The position of the first quartile is $0.25 \times 12 = 3$
  - Rounding up, the first quartile is the value at the third position, which is 26.
- Calculate the Third Quartile (75th Percentile):
  - The position of the third quartile is $0.75 \times 12 = 9$
  - Rounding up, the third quartile is the value at the ninth position, which is 38.

The median (50th percentile) is 33, indicating that 50% of the patients have a BMI of 33 or lower. The first quartile (25th percentile) is 26, meaning that 25% of the patients have a BMI of 26 or lower. The third quartile (75th percentile) is 38, suggesting that 75% of the patients have a BMI of 38 or lower. These percentiles provide insights into the distribution of BMI values within the sample of 12 patients.

Standard Deviation

The standard deviation is the most commonly reported measure of variability, and it is derived from deviations of values from the mean in a given dataset. While the mean represents the expected average of the data set, the standard deviation quantifies the average deviations of values from the mean. Whenever a mean is reported, it is essential to include the corresponding standard deviation. This measure, based on the normal curve, helps determine the number of data values falling within specific intervals in a normal distribution.

Understanding the standard deviation enables the interpretation of an individual score in relation to all other scores in the dataset. Referring back to the earlier example of heart rates given in Table 2.4, the data exhibited variability due to the wide range of heart rate values. Calculating the standard deviation provides distinct information about this variability. It becomes evident that the average deviation from the mean for the experimental group is 11.36, more than of the control group, which has a deviation of 7.47.

Confidence Interval

A confidence interval (CI) serves as a statistical method for approximating the potential range in which a population parameter, such as the mean or proportion, is probable to be situated. This estimation is derived from a sample of data and offers insight into the uncertainty linked with the estimate. Typically presented as a range around a point estimate, confidence intervals convey the degree of confidence in the likelihood that the actual population parameter falls within that specified range.

Confidence intervals are typically portrayed as a span around a central point estimate, like the mean, and the width of the interval signifies the extent of uncertainty. While the 95% confidence interval is widely employed, it is feasible to compute intervals at different confidence levels, such as 90% or 99%. The endpoints of the confidence interval are referred to as limits or bounds.

For example, in Table 2.2, which details the heart rates of 50 patients, the sample mean heart rate was 78.88, and the standard deviation was 6.65. The calculations for the confidence intervals (CI) for the mean heart rate at different confidence levels are as follows:

– *95% confidence interval:*
  First the *t*-value ($df = 49$) ≈ 2.009

$$\text{Margin of Error}_{95\%} = 2.009 \times \left(\frac{6.65}{\sqrt{50}} \right) \approx 1.784$$

$$CI_{95\%} = 78.88 \pm 1.784$$

The 95% confidence interval for the heart rate is approximately [77.10, 80.66].

– *99% confidence interval:*
  First the *t*-value ($df = 49$) ≈ 2.281

$$\text{Margin of Error}_{99\%} = 2.281 \times \left(\frac{6.65}{\sqrt{50}} \right) \approx 2.389$$

$$CI_{99\%} = 78.88 \pm 2.389$$

The 99% confidence interval for the heart rate is approximately [76.49, 81.27].

– *90% confidence interval:*
  First the *t*-value ($df = 49$) ≈ 1.684

$$\text{Margin of Error}_{90\%} = 1.684 \times \left(\frac{6.65}{\sqrt{50}} \right) \approx 1.501$$

$$CI_{90\%} = 78.88 \pm 1.501$$

The 90% confidence interval for the heart rate is approximately [77.38, 80.38].

Understanding confidence intervals is crucial in statistical analysis as they provide a more comprehensive perspective than a singular point estimate. The choice of a specific confidence level (95%, 99%, or 90%) involves a trade-off between the width of the interval and the level of certainty. They allow researchers and analysts to gauge the precision of their estimates and convey the inherent variability in the data. Additionally, confidence intervals facilitate informed decision-making by offering a sense of the potential range of values for the population parameter under consideration.

Standard Score

A standard score is a measurement employed to assess how far an observation, such as a test score, deviates from the mean of a population or sample, expressed in standard deviation units. Standard scores provide a means to identify the position of a given score within the bell curve or frequency distribution concerning the comparison population or sample.

By converting raw scores into standard scores, one gains insights into how a particular observation stands relative to the average and variability of the dataset. Positive and negative values indicate whether a score is above or below the mean, respectively. This standardized approach facilitates a more uniform and interpretable comparison of scores across different distributions, enabling a clearer understanding of the relative positioning of individual observations within the broader context of the data.

2.5.2.6 Normal Distribution

However, data often deviate from normal distribution, becoming skewed or asymmetric. In asymmetric distributions, the data peak is not centered, and one tail is longer Fig. 2.6c. Negative skewness, depicted in Fig. 2.6a with a leftward tail, occurs when the mean is less than the median and mode. This results from a lower score pulling down the mean and influencing the leftward tail.

For example, in a clinical nursing student assessment, most show competent performance, but a few struggles with certain aspects, causing lower scores. This creates a negatively skewed distribution, with the mean score pulled down by the struggling students, resulting in a longer left tail. The majority performs adequately, but the presence of struggling individuals contributes to the leftward skewness.

Conversely, positive skewness, pulling the tail to the right, occurs when the mean is greater than the median and mode (Fig. 2.6b). For example, in an evaluation of experienced clinical nurses, most perform at a high level, providing standard care. However, a few excel with extraordinary skills in handling challenging cases, creating a positively skewed distribution. The mean skill level is elevated by these outstanding performers, resulting in a rightward-tailed distribution. While most nurses demonstrate proficiency, the presence of exceptionally skilled individuals contributes to the rightward skewness.

Examining data dispersion around the mean is crucial. Uniform data, akin to individuals in uniforms, show minimal spread and a cohesive appearance. Increased variability leads to a wider spread in data. Graphically, highly uniform data display a tall peak, while highly variable data exhibit a lower peak. Kurtosis, the term for a data set's peakiness or flatness, captures this characteristic.

2.5.2.7 Tailedness

Understanding the concept of tailedness is crucial in statistical analysis. A normal distribution, characterized by symmetrical data with the mean, median, and mode all equal, is typically represented by a bell-shaped curve centered around the mean (x). This distribution extends up to three

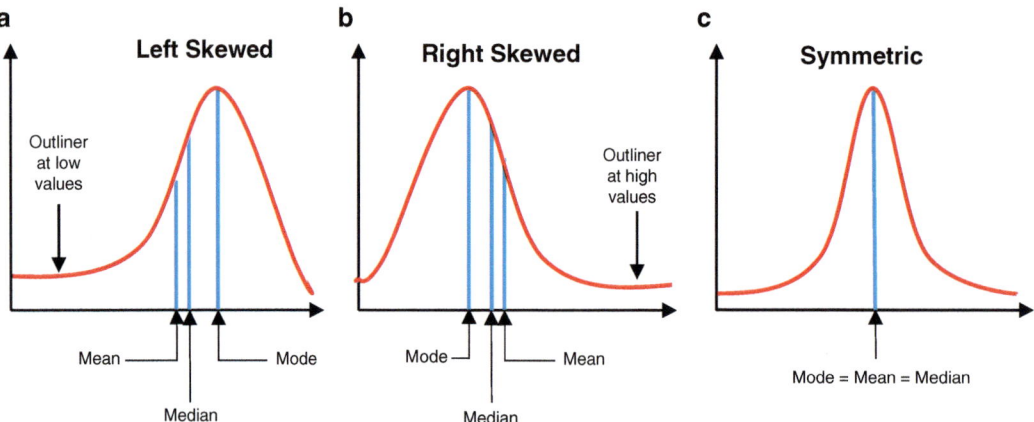

Fig. 2.6 (**a**) Skewed to the left (left-skewed): The mean and median are less than the mode. (**b**) Skewed to the right (right skewed): The mean and median are greater than the mode. (**c**) Symmetric distribution: The mean, median, and mode are the same

standard deviations on both the positive and negative sides. Approximately, 99.7% of data points fall within this range, with 68.3% within one standard deviation and 95.5% within two standard deviations of the mean, as outlined in the Rule of 68.3 –95.5 –99.7 Fig. 2.7.

The symmetry of the normal distribution is evident in the division of standard deviations, with each containing a proportion of data above and below the mean. For instance, one standard deviation encompasses 34.13% of scores above and below the mean, totaling 68.3%, while two standard deviations include 34.13% plus 13.6% above and below the mean, summing up to 95.5% of scores Fig. 2.7. The mean on a standard deviation graph is represented by a z-score of zero, and other z-score percentages can be determined using tables showing the area under the curve.

In a normal distribution, the significance level pertains to specific areas in the tails of the curve. In a one-tailed test Fig. 2.8, the entire significance level is assigned to either the left or right tail of the distribution. For instance, with a significance level of 0.05 (5%), if your data point falls within the 5% tail on one side of the distribution, you would reject the null hypothesis. To clarify, a right-tailed test involves rejecting the null hypothesis if the data point falls in the upper 5% tail, while a left-tailed test does so for the lower 5% tail. In this scenario, if the observed value is statistically significant ($p \leq 0.05$), the null hypothesis (H_0) is dismissed, and the alternative hypothesis (H_a) is embraced. This implies that there's enough evidence to support the alternative hypothesis over the null hypothesis.

In a normal distribution, the significance level is associated with specific segments in the tails of the curve. In a two-tailed test Fig. 2.9, these segments each encompass 2.5% of the total area under the curve. If any data point falls within these extreme regions, it would be deemed statistically significant at the 0.05 level, prompting rejection of the null hypothesis. Essentially, for a two-tailed test, both ends of the distribution are considered, and any deviation in either direction from the expected values could lead to rejecting

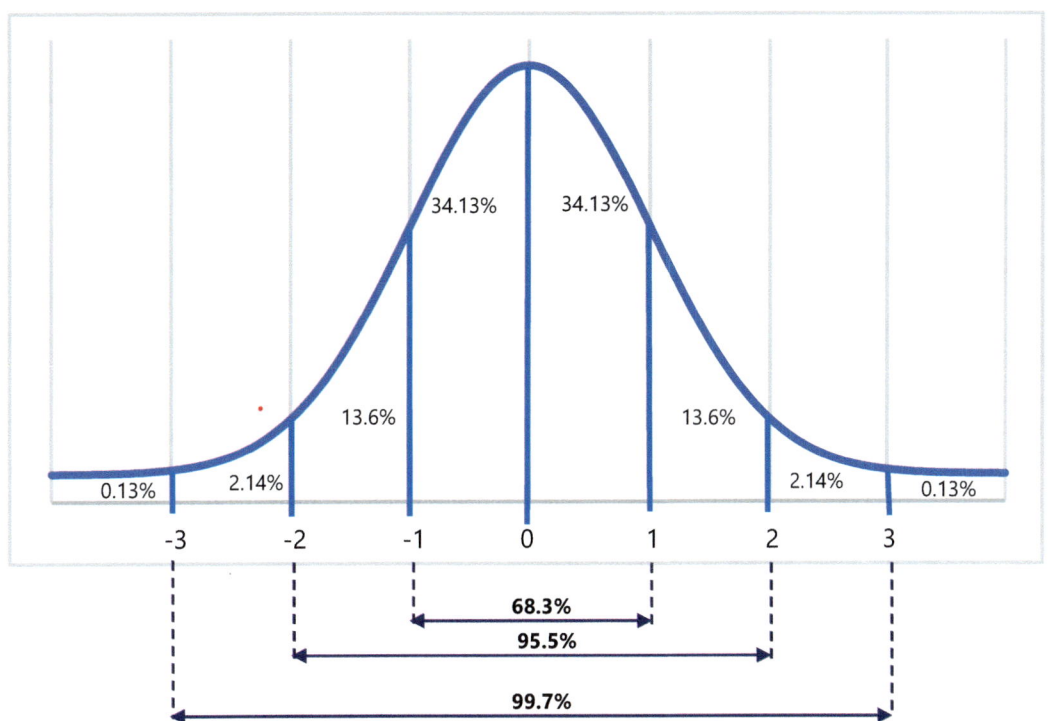

Fig. 2.7 Normal distribution and percentage of data within the standard deviation from the mean

Fig. 2.8 One- tailed test of 0.05 level of significance

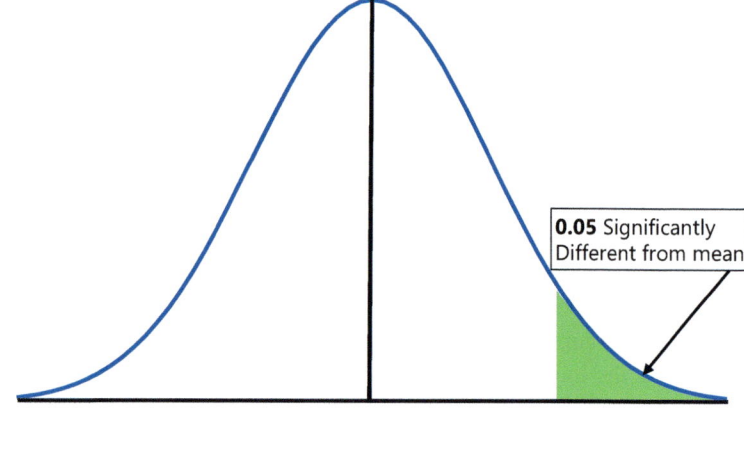

0.05 Significantly Different from mean

Fig. 2.9 Two- tailed test of 0.05 level of significance

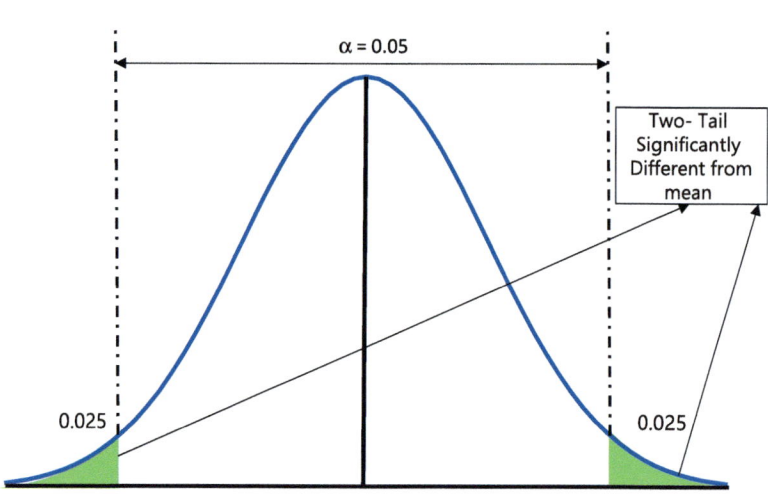

$\alpha = 0.05$

Two- Tail Significantly Different from mean

0.025

0.025

the null hypothesis in favor of the alternative. This ensures thorough examination for significant deviations in either direction from the expected outcome.

2.5.2.8 Type I and Type II Errors

The process of determining whether to accept or reject a null hypothesis is crucial in assessing the likelihood that observed group differences are merely due to chance, especially considering the incomplete knowledge researchers have about the population. Consequently, statistical inferences inherently entail a degree of uncertainty and the risk of error. Two primary types of errors can arise: Type I, where researchers incorrectly reject a true null hypothesis, and Type II, where researchers mistakenly accept a false null hypothesis [13]. Type I errors occur when researchers reject the null hypothesis despite its truth. For example, if researchers conclude that a particular postoperative pain management technique is more effective in reducing pain compared to a standard approach, when in reality, observed differences are due to random fluctuations in the sample, it constitutes a Type I error. Conversely, Type II errors arise when researchers mistakenly accept a false null hypothesis. If researchers attribute differences in pain scores to chance when the intervention actually reduces pain, it signifies a Type II error.

2.5.3 Inferential Statistics

Several factors influence the appropriateness of using inferential statistical methods in a study.

These methods are employed to explore relationships, make predictions, and ascertain causality or discrepancies in research. Assessing statistical procedures necessitates making various judgments regarding the data's nature and the researcher's objectives. Key considerations include: (1) The research question or hypothesis; (2) The data's level of measurement (nominal, ordinal, or interval/ratio); (3) The number of groups involved; and (4) Whether the groups are paired (dependent) or independent [14].

In a study investigating the effectiveness of a new pain management intervention for postoperative patients, researchers may employ both independent and paired groups. Patients randomly assigned to receive either the new intervention or standard care represent independent groups. However, for paired groups, researchers might use a pretest–posttest design, where each patient serves as their own control. For instance, patients' pain levels are measured before and after receiving the intervention. Additionally, researchers may match pairs of patients based on factors such as age, type of surgery, or preoperative pain severity to minimize the influence of these variables.

2.5.3.1 Parametric and Nonparametric Tests

Statistical tests can be broadly classified into two categories. *Parametric tests*, which are more commonly used by researchers, possess three defining characteristics: (1) they involve estimating a parameter; (2) they necessitate measurements on at least an interval scale; and (3) they rely on various assumptions, including the assumption of normality in the variables' distribution within the population.

In contrast, *nonparametric tests* do not involve parameter estimation. They are typically employed when data are measured on a nominal or ordinal scale. Nonparametric methods have less stringent assumptions regarding the shape of the variables' distribution compared to parametric tests. Consequently, nonparametric tests are sometimes referred to as distribution-free statistics.

Parametric tests are generally more statistically powerful than nonparametric tests and are often preferred. However, there exists some disagreement regarding the appropriateness of nonparametric tests. Some purists argue that if the prerequisites for parametric tests are not met, nonparametric tests should not be used. Nevertheless, numerous statistical studies suggest that violating the assumptions of parametric tests does not significantly affect statistical decision-making.

A more moderate viewpoint in this debate, which we find reasonable, is that nonparametric tests are particularly useful when data cannot be interpreted as interval-level or when the distribution significantly deviates from normality. Given the importance of selecting appropriate statistical analysis techniques, it is essential to understand the distinctions between parametric and nonparametric tests as well as how to determine the most suitable method for a given research study.

One method for assessing the suitability of an analysis technique in a study involves using a decision tree or algorithm. This algorithm guides the user by progressively narrowing down the range of appropriate analysis techniques as judgments are made regarding the study's nature and the data it involves. In the flowchart shown in Fig. 2.10, a variety of tests are utilized to analyze data with the objective of determining whether there is a statistically significant difference, relationship, or predictor analysis between the groups [15]. Researchers must consider the number of groups to be included in the analysis and the level at which variables were measured when deciding which test to use.

2.5.3.2 Examining Differences

Inferential statistics serve as a powerful tool for scrutinizing disparities between groups, such as assessing variances between intervention and control groups across selected demographic variables. These statistical methods are not only instrumental in identifying causality of the independent variable on the dependent variable but also offer a means of understanding how one event influences or triggers another. Analytical

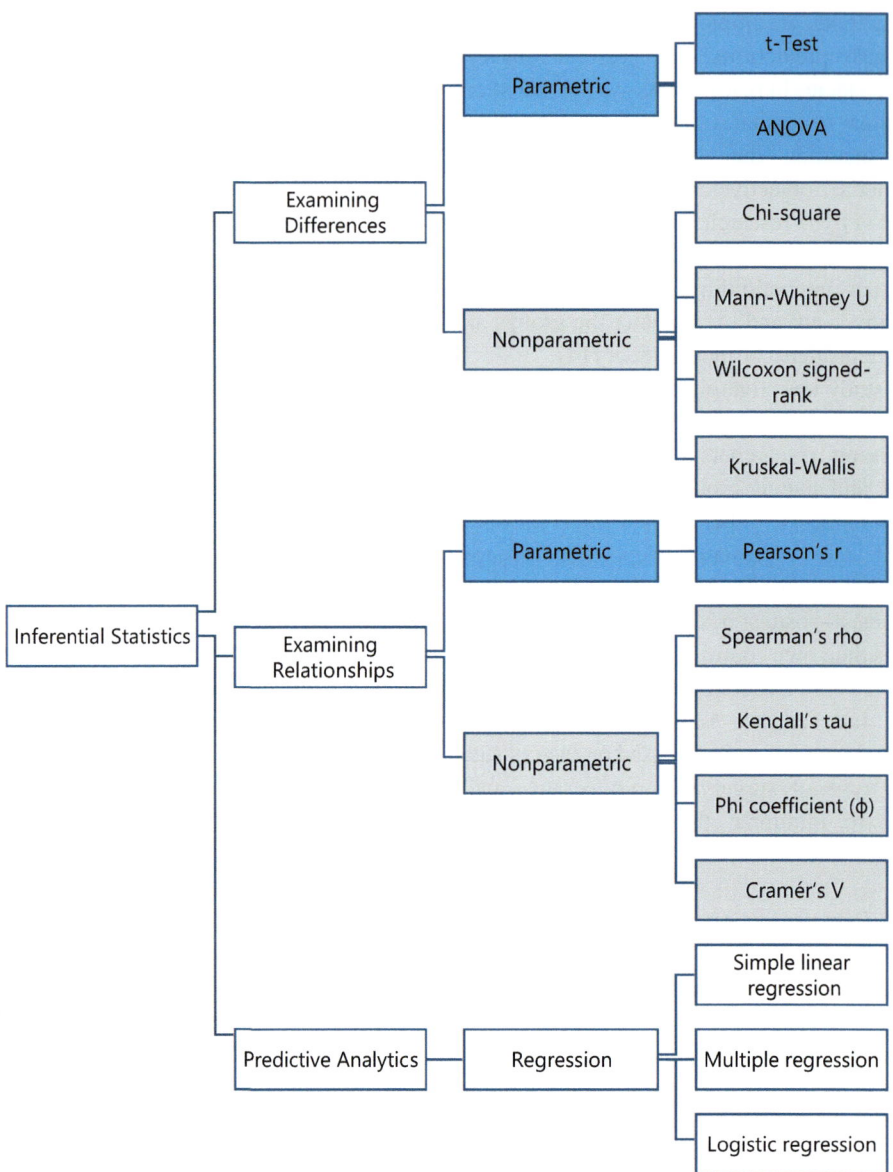

Fig. 2.10 Decision tree for selecting inferential statistical tests

techniques aimed at examining causality play a crucial role in discerning the impacts of interventions on patient and family outcomes.

Various statistical procedures are employed to examine differences, including the *t*-test, analysis of variance (ANOVA), and analysis of covariance (ANCOVA). The *t*-test, specifically, is adept at discerning discrepancies between two groups, while the chi-square test, ANOVA, and ANCOVA are adept at exploring differences among three or more groups. Furthermore, the chi-square test is tailored for analyzing nominal or ordinal data levels, whereas the *t*-test, ANOVA, and ANCOVA are suited for analyzing interval and ratio data levels. These diverse statistical approaches collectively facilitate a comprehensive examination of differences across various research contexts.

For example, researchers might conduct a study to compare the effectiveness of two pain management approaches in postoperative patients. One group would receive traditional pain medications, while the other group would undergo a non-pharmacological intervention, such as acupuncture. Through this research setup, the study aims to assess whether acupuncture provides comparable or better pain relief than standard medication. Using inferential statistics, such as t-tests or ANOVA, researchers can analyze the differences in pain levels between the two groups, thus determining the efficacy of acupuncture as an alternative pain management strategy for postoperative patients. By scrutinizing significant differences in outcomes between intervention and control groups, these statistics provide valuable insights into the effectiveness of interventions.

2.5.3.3 Chi-Square Test

The chi-square test is utilized to ascertain whether two variables are independent or correlated, and it can be applied to nominal or ordinal data. This procedure involves examining the observed frequencies of data values and comparing them with the expected frequencies under the assumption of independence between the variables. The chi-square (χ^2) test is a nonparametric procedure used to test hypotheses about the proportion of cases that fall into different categories, as when a contingency table has been created. However, this test is not particularly robust, leading to a high risk of Type II error, where the study fails to detect significant differences even if they truly exist. To mitigate this risk, large sample sizes are often required. Moreover, in many studies employing this test, little emphasis is placed on results where no differences are detected. Researchers frequently conduct multiple chi-square tests within a sample, but typically only report significant differences identified through these analyses.

For example, in analyzing the association between nurse staffing levels and patient falls, researchers relied on the calculated Chi-square statistic, degrees of freedom, and the chosen alpha level to consult Chi-square tables for determining the critical value and evaluating its statistical significance. In scholarly literature, Chi-square notations such as $\chi^2 = 1.89$, $df = 1$,

$p < 0.05$ are commonly reported alongside degrees of freedom and significance. Chi-square tests are preferred for their computational simplicity, obviating the need for advanced statistical software. However, it is essential to ensure an adequate sample size, with each cell in the table containing at least five observed frequencies. Failure to meet this criterion necessitates using Fisher's exact probability test as an alternative to Chi-square.

t-Test

The t statistic, commonly referred to as the t-test or Student's t-test, is frequently reported in nursing research. This parametric measure serves to determine whether a statistically significant difference exists between two groups. The t-test is widely utilized to examine group disparities when variables are measured at the interval or ratio levels. Different types of t-tests have been developed to suit various sample scenarios: for independent groups, researchers apply the t-test for independent samples, while for paired or dependent groups, the t-test for paired samples is utilized.

However, misuse of the t-test is not uncommon among researchers, particularly when conducting multiple comparisons on different aspects of collected data. Such misuse can lead to an escalation of significance, heightening the risk of a Type I error—erroneously concluding significance where none exists. To address this issue, the Bonferroni procedure is often employed, adjusting the significance level based on the number of comparisons conducted.

For example, in a study investigating anxiety levels among nurses during night shifts, participants could be divided into two groups based on their experience: those with over 2 years and those with less than 2 years of experience. The t-test was conducted to compare anxiety levels among nurses during night shifts based on their experience levels. Participants were divided into two groups: those with over 2 years of experience ($n = 50$) and those with less than 2 years of experience ($n = 40$). The mean anxiety level for nurses with over 2 years of experience was $M = 3.8$ (SD = 1.2), whereas for nurses with less than

2 years of experience, it was $M = 4.5$ (SD = 1.5). The t-test revealed a statistically significant difference in anxiety levels between the two groups (t (88) = −2.36, $p < 0.05$), indicating that experience level significantly impacts anxiety during night shifts.

Nonparametric Alternatives to t-Test

In situations where t-tests may not be appropriate, particularly in scenarios involving two groups with ordinal scale dependent variables or significantly non-normal distributions, nonparametric tests provide alternative methods. One such method is the *Mann-Whitney U test,* which assesses differences between two independent groups when the dependent variable is measured on an ordinal scale. This test entails assigning ranks to measures from both groups, and then comparing the sum of the ranks for each group using the U statistic. The Mann-Whitney U test is considered more powerful than the median test as it retains more information.

For paired (dependent) ordinal-level data, researchers have options such as the sign test and the *Wilcoxon signed-rank test.* The sign test involves assigning a positive or negative symbol to score differences based on whether one score is larger than the other. Conversely, the Wilcoxon signed-rank test involves calculating the difference between paired scores, ranking the absolute differences, and then evaluating the ranks.

While nonparametric tests offer computational simplicity compared to t-tests, it is crucial to avoid selecting a statistical method solely based on ease of computation, particularly when computerized analysis tools are available.

Analysis of Variance (ANOVA)

Analysis of Variance (ANOVA) serves as a statistical tool when dealing with interval or ratio level measurements and involves more than two groups or multiple measurements of the variable of interest [16, 17]. Its primary aim is to determine if there are significant differences among group means. Employing ANOVA enables researchers to compare various pairs of means simultaneously, thus minimizing the likelihood of a type I error. For instance, consider a scenario where a nurse researcher investigates the effectiveness of three different pain management techniques among postoperative patients: pharmacological, acupuncture, and relaxation therapy. Comparing all possible pairs of means—pharmacological vs. acupuncture, pharmacological vs. relaxation therapy, and acupuncture vs. relaxation therapy—through separate t-tests would increase the risk of committing a type I error threefold. By opting for ANOVA, nurse researchers can assess variations in pain management effectiveness using a single statistical test, thereby mitigating the risk of erroneously concluding significant differences.

Analysis of Variance (ANOVA) and t-tests are closely related statistical methods. When comparing only two groups, both ANOVA and t-tests yield the same result mathematically. However, ANOVA offers the advantage of calculating the F statistic, which is based on the F distribution using degrees of freedom. A higher F statistic indicates greater variation among group means. For instance, a notation like $F = 4.65$, $df = 2, 50$, $p < 0.05$ may be used to report ANOVA results. Nonetheless, while the F statistic indicates a rejection of the null hypothesis due to differences between group means, it does not specify which group differs significantly. To identify the specific group(s) with significant differences, researchers often conduct post hoc tests.

Two variations of ANOVA, namely analysis of covariance (ANCOVA) and multivariate analysis of variance (MANOVA), play essential roles in nursing research. ANCOVA serves the purpose of statistically controlling for known extraneous variables, enhancing the accuracy of research findings. For instance, a researcher aims to assess how different pain management techniques impact the recovery outcomes of postoperative patients. In such cases, ANCOVA could be utilized to control for various pre-existing factors related to pain management, such as comorbidities. By incorporating these variables as covariates, ANCOVA enables researchers to isolate the specific influence of the pain management technique on recovery outcomes, while simultaneously considering the potential effects of confounding factors.

Conversely, in studies involving multiple dependent variables associated with pain management outcomes, such as pain intensity, functional ability, and psychological well-being, researchers may opt for MANOVA over ANOVA. This choice allows for a more comprehensive analysis that accounts for the interrelationships among these variables. By employing MANOVA, researchers can gain a deeper understanding of the complex interactions between various aspects of pain management and patient outcomes, thereby enriching the depth and breadth of their research findings.

Nonparametric Alternatives to Analysis of Variance

Nonparametric methods, while not specifically analyzing variance, offer alternatives to ANOVA when dealing with ordinal-level data or highly non-normal distributions where parametric tests are not suitable. One such method is the *Kruskal-Wallis test*, which serves as a generalized version of the Mann-Whitney U test. This test involves assigning ranks to scores across different groups and is applicable when there are more than two groups and a one-way test for independent samples is required. Additionally, when multiple measures are obtained from the same subjects, the Friedman test provides a nonparametric approach for "analysis of variance" by ranks.

2.5.3.4 Examining Relationships

Researchers utilize correlational analyses to explore connections between variables, aiming to describe, clarify, or potentially uncover causal relationships. These analyses require data from a single population, ensuring availability of values for all variables under investigation. For robust insights into the nature of relationships, data measured at the interval or ratio level are preferred, offering more detailed information.

2.5.3.5 Pearson's r

Researchers utilize correlational analyses to explore relationships between variables, aiming to describe, clarify, or identify causal relationships. These analyses require data from a single population and are most informative when vari-

ables are measured at the interval or ratio level. Pearson's r, also known as the Pearson product–moment correlation, is employed when testing hypotheses concerning variable relationships, particularly when variables are measured at the interval or ratio level. Traditionally, correlation coefficients below ±0.3 are deemed weak, those between ±0.3 and ±0.5 are considered moderate, and values exceeding ±0.5 are categorized as strong relationships. However, interpretation should be nuanced, considering factors such as variable characteristics and measurement context. Correlational analyses yield symmetrical outcomes, indicating that they do not reveal the direction of the relationship between variables. Symmetrical outcomes mean that it is impossible to determine from the analysis whether variable A influences or causes variable B, or vice versa. Correlational analysis techniques primarily focus on exploring relationships between variables rather than establishing cause-and-effect relationships.

The coefficient's square (r^2) reveals the percentage of variance explained by the relationship, aiding in understanding the extent to which variables predict each other's values. Despite a strong correlation, variables may not perfectly align, as indicated by the variance unexplained by the relationship. Understanding and interpreting Pearson's r correlation coefficients necessitates a nuanced approach, considering both statistical significance and practical implications within the context of the study.

Nonparametric Test to Measure the Relationship

In situations where the assumptions for parametric tests are not met or when dealing with ordinal-level data, alternative correlation coefficients such as Spearman's rho (rS) or Kendall's tau are more appropriate. Unlike Pearson's r, which relies on the assumption of normality and linearity, *Spearman's rho* and *Kendall's tau* are nonparametric measures of association that do not require these assumptions.

Spearman's rho is calculated by ranking the data and then computing the Pearson correlation coefficient for the ranks. It measures the strength and direction of the monotonic relationship between two variables, where monotonicity implies that as one variable increases, the other variable either consistently increases or decreases.

Kendall's tau, on the other hand, assesses the strength and direction of association between two variables based on the number of concordant and discordant pairs in the data. It is particularly useful when dealing with tied ranks or when analyzing ordinal data with small sample sizes.

In addition to these correlation coefficients, measures of relationship magnitude can be calculated for nominal-level data. For instance, the *phi coefficient* (ϕ) quantifies the relationship between two dichotomous variables by comparing observed and expected frequencies. A high phi coefficient indicates a strong association between the variables.

Similarly, *Cramér's V* is applied to contingency tables larger than 2×2 and assesses the strength of association between categorical variables. It is computed by taking the square root of the chi-square statistic divided by the total number of observations or the minimum of the number of rows minus 1 and the number of columns minus 1. Cramér's *V* ranges between 0 and 1, with higher values indicating stronger associations between variables.

2.5.3.6 Predictive Analytics

The ability to forecast future events is increasingly crucial worldwide, including in nursing practice. Nurse researchers, like others in society, rely on predictive abilities. For example, they aim to anticipate factors affecting wound healing, such as oxygenation, infection, age, sex hormones, stress, diabetes, obesity, medications, alcoholism, smoking, and nutrition. They seek to predict how these elements will influence the healing process in patients with wounds of varying severity and characteristics. A deeper understanding of these factors' influence on repair may lead to therapeutic interventions that enhance wound healing and resolve impaired wounds. Such advancements not only reduce treatment costs but also improve the patient's overall well-being. Predictive analyses are grounded in prob-

ability theory rather than decision theory, providing a means to explore causal relationships among variables.

2.5.3.7 Regression Analysis

Regression analysis serves to predict one variable's value when the values of one or more other variables are known. The variable to be predicted is termed the dependent or outcome variable, typically measured at the interval or ratio level. The analysis aims to explain as much variance in the dependent variable as possible, with the predictors referred to as independent variables.

Simple linear regression is utilized in nursing research when investigating the relationship between a single independent variable and a dependent variable. For instance, researchers might employ simple linear regression to explore whether there is a linear relationship between the number of nursing staff available and patient satisfaction scores. In this example, the independent variable would be the number of nursing staff, while the dependent variable would be patient satisfaction scores. The researchers would hypothesize that patients who experience more interaction with nursing staff throughout their hospitalization tend to report higher satisfaction scores.

Multiple regression analyses data with two or more independent variables, allowing researchers to investigate the combined effects of these variables on a dependent variable. For example, multiple regression could be used to examine how patient satisfaction scores are influenced by factors such as the number of nursing staff, the availability of medical equipment, the cleanliness of the hospital environment and patient age. In this example, the independent variables would be the number of nursing staff, availability of medical equipment, cleanliness of the hospital environment, and patient age while the dependent variable would still be patient satisfaction scores. Researchers would hypothesize that these multiple factors collectively impact patient satisfaction, rather than any single factor alone.

Dependent and independent variables are symbolized by *Y* and *X*, respectively. Prior to regression analysis, scatterplots and correlation matrices are often created to explore variable relationships Fig. 2.11. The analysis seeks to establish a line of best fit reflecting scatterplot values, commonly visualized as an overlay.

Various regression techniques, including logistic regression, have been developed to analyze diverse data types. *Logistic regression*, increasingly used to predicts values of a nominal-level dependent variable, assessing patient response to interventions.

The outcome of regression analysis is the regression coefficient, denoted as R. R^2 signifies the proportion of variance in the data explained by the equation and is termed the coefficient of multiple determination when multiple independent variables are used. Test statistics like t or F determine the significance of regression coefficients, with small sample sizes reducing statistical significance likelihood. Reports include R^2 and t (from t-test) or F (from the analysis of variance [ANOVA]) values, but understanding complex regression results necessitates careful reading, term lookup, and statistical significance assessment.

2.5.4   Factor Analysis

Factor analysis, commonly employed in psychology and education, is instrumental in interpreting self-reporting questionnaires. This statistical method offers numerous advantages, such as condensing multiple variables into a smaller set of factors and revealing underlying dimensions between measured variables and latent constructs [18]. Additionally, factor analysis provides evidence of construct validity for self-reporting scales.

There are two primary types of factor analysis: exploratory factor analysis (EFA) and confirmatory factor analysis (CFA). EFA, operating without preconceived notions, explores dimensions to generate theories from latent constructs. Conversely, CFA tests pre-existing theories, guided by prior assumptions regarding factor numbers and fit.

For example, a researcher eager to assess job satisfaction among nurses across various hospital departments. They administer a comprehensive survey comprising 50 questions covering multiple aspects of job satisfaction. Rather than ana-

Fig. 2.11 Example for scatterplot for best fit line

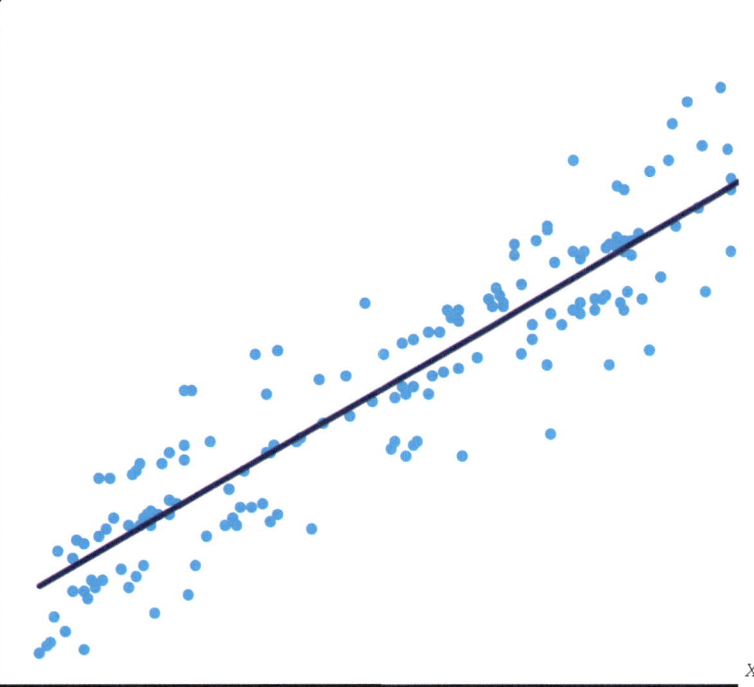

lyzing each of the 50 questions independently, the researcher opts for exploratory factor analysis (EFA) to identify underlying dimensions contributing to job satisfaction. Through this process, they uncover factors like workload, work environment dynamics, support mechanisms, opportunities for growth, and recognition. For instance, the workload dimension might include questions related to the number of patients attended to daily, while the work environment dynamics factor could encompass questions about the quality of teamwork. Support mechanisms may be assessed through questions about access to mentorship programs, while opportunities for growth could involve queries regarding access to continuing education. Recognition might be evaluated through questions about acknowledgment of achievements. This structured approach simplifies analysis while providing a deeper understanding of job satisfaction's multifaceted nature in nursing.

Building on the findings from EFA, the researcher develops a theoretical model postulating relationships between observed variables and latent constructs. For instance, they hypothesize that workload and work environment contribute to "Work Satisfaction," while support from colleagues and supervisors forms "Social Satisfaction." Administering the survey to a new sample, the researcher conducts CFA to evaluate the model fit. Statistical indices like Comparative Fit Index (CFI) and Root Mean Square Error of Approximation (RMSEA) are used for assessment. A satisfactory fit substantiates the theoretical framework, enhancing confidence in understanding job satisfaction among nurses. Conversely, poor fit prompts model refinement or exploration of alternative explanations, underscoring CFA's role in validating theoretical constructs.

2.6   Validity and Reliability

Validating and ensuring the reliability of research findings are integral to upholding research quality standards [19]. In nursing practice, the utiliza-

tion of evidence from well-executed research is fundamental. Thus, the ability to assess quantitative research critically is an essential skill for nurses. Beyond scrutinizing study outcomes, attention must be paid to the rigor of the research process. Rigor, in this context, pertains to the efforts made by researchers to enhance study quality, notably through the measurement of validity and reliability in quantitative research (Fig. 2.12).

2.6.1   Measurement Error

Measurement error is an inherent aspect of any measurement process, representing the variance between the true measure and the actual measurement obtained. This error can vary significantly from one measurement to another, even in supposedly precise direct measures. In healthcare, efforts to evaluate various parameters often face challenges due to measurement inaccuracies. The overarching goal of any measurement is to align the observed measurement as closely as possible with the true measurement. This relationship is represented by the equation:

$$O = T + E,$$

where O signifies the observed score obtained from the instrument, and T represents the true score, reflecting the actual amount of the characteristic being measured. Ideally, if O equals T, it would indicate a perfect instrument, but in practice, error (E) is always present during measurements. This error can manifest as either random error or systematic error. Error can appear in the form of either random error or systematic error.

Random error refers to error that arises by chance and is challenging for researchers to control because it stems from transient factors. This type of error can be attributed to various factors such as subject characteristics, variations in instrumentation, or environmental conditions. For instance, a nurse is assessing pain levels in a patient following surgery. Despite a patient accurately describes moderate pain to a nurse, but due to miscommunication or misunderstanding, the nurse records a lower pain score. As a result, the

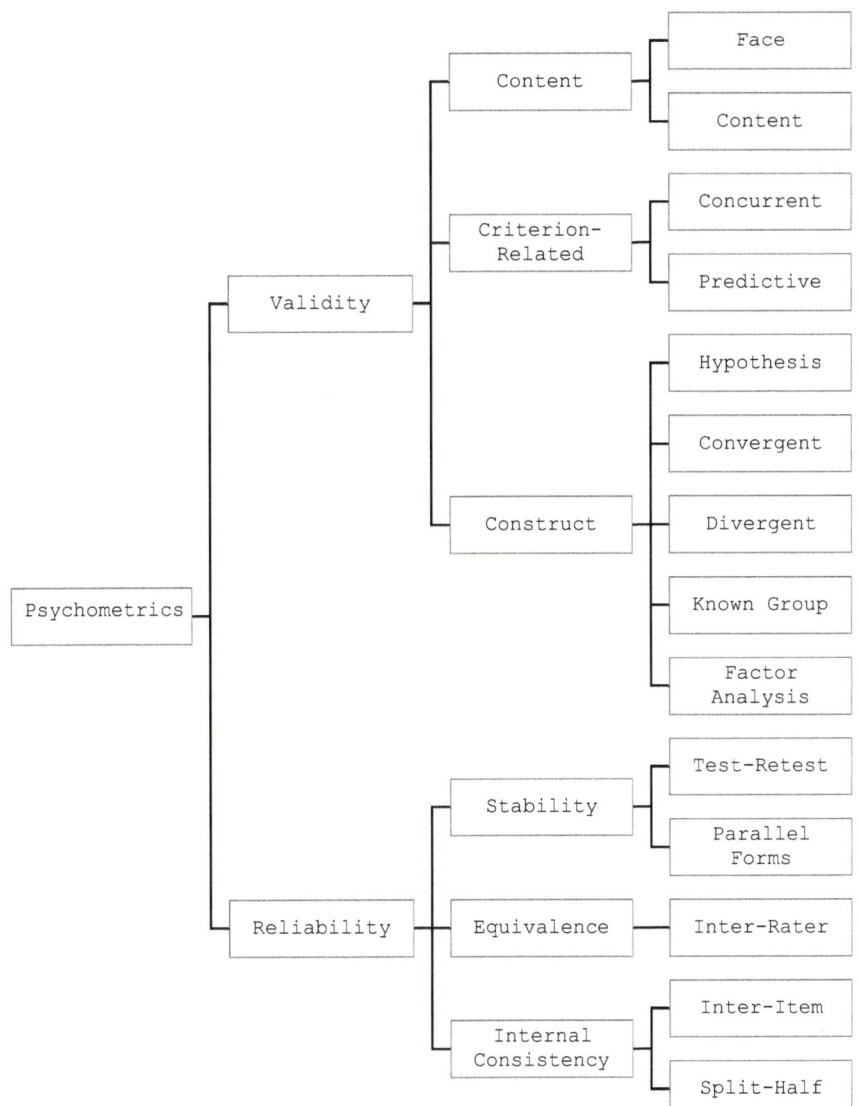

Fig. 2.12 Types of reliability and validity in qualitative research

observed pain level appears lower than the patient's true level of pain.

On the other hand, systematic error occurs when the same type of error consistently repeats. Also referred to as consistent error, it can arise from factors related to subjects, instrumentation, or the environment. For example, a researcher measures body temperatures following an intervention using an electronic thermometer assumed to be accurate. However, if the thermometer has not been calibrated recently, it may consistently report temperatures half a degree lower than the actual values. This error affects every temperature measurement, making it systematic in nature.

In the context of *psychometrics*, the presence of error in measurement is a fundamental consideration. Psychometricians recognize that measurement error is inevitable and strive to minimize its impact on the validity and reliability of psychological measures. They employ rigorous methodologies to develop and evaluate measurement instruments, taking into account the potential sources of error and implementing strategies to mitigate them. By acknowledging the inherent error in measurement, psychometricians aim to enhance the accuracy and precision of psychological assessment tools. Through techniques such as *factor analysis*, item response theory, and classical test theory, they seek to understand and quantify the extent of measurement error and its effects on the validity and reliability of measurement instruments.

Moreover, the field of psychometrics emphasizes the importance of transparency and rigor in measurement practices. Researchers are encouraged to document and report on the psychometric properties of their instruments, including evidence of *validity, reliability*, and any potential sources of error. Overall, recognizing and addressing measurement error is central to the field of psychometrics, as it ensures that psychological measures are valid, reliable, and fair representations of the constructs they intend to assess.

2.6.2 Validity

In quantitative studies, validity refers to the accuracy of measuring a concept, guiding researchers when selecting instruments to ensure their validity. Validity reflects how well an instrument captures the intended measurement, such as in clinical nursing, where nurses must choose tools accurately measuring postoperative pain, distinguishing it from related factors like anxiety or discomfort. Validity includes three types: content validity, criterion-related validity, and construct validity, each crucial for ensuring accurate measurement in research [20].

2.6.2.1 Content Validity
Content validity is achieved when researchers confirm that the instrument accurately measures the intended concept, necessitating a clear definition of the studied concept to ensure alignment with the selected instrument. This validation process involves two approaches: *face validity* and *content validity* testing, both of which entail external evaluation of the instruments. While face validity relies on subjective judgments from colleagues or subjects, content validity testing engages expert panels to assess each item's alignment with the measured concept. Based on panel feedback, researchers refine the instrument by retaining items with high ratings and modifying or eliminating those with low ratings. For example, in the development of the Pittsburgh Sleep Quality Index (PSQI), researchers involved participants in rating various aspects of sleep quality, such as sleep latency and disturbances. This collaboration allowed for the refinement of the scale based on participants' experiences and perceptions, ensuring its relevance and accuracy in assessing sleep quality.

2.6.2.2 Criterion-Related Validity
Criterion-related validity assesses the relationship between the observed score and the true score. Researchers typically examine this validity through *concurrent validity* and *predictive validity*. Concurrent validity involves comparing a new instrument with an already established valid instrument that measures the same concept, using correlation analysis to determine agreement. Conversely, predictive validity evaluates whether scores obtained at one point in time correlate with scores obtained at a future time point. For example, if researchers are developing a depression screening tool, they might assess its criterion-related validity by comparing it to an established measure of depression. If the new tool demonstrates a strong correlation with the established measure, it suggests good concurrent validity. Additionally, they could assess predictive validity by administering the screening tool to a group of individuals and then following up with them after 6 months to see if those who scored high on the screening tool were more likely to develop clinical depression.

2.6.2.3 Construct Validity
Construct validity is centered on theoretical concepts, known as constructs, which are empirically tested. Researchers assess how well an instrument measures these theoretical constructs.

Establishing construct validity necessitates sophisticated strategies and prolonged empirical testing. To establish construct validity, researchers utilize various methods including *hypothesis testing, convergent testing, divergent testing, known group testing,* and *factor analysis.*

In *hypothesis testing*, researchers utilize theories to predict outcomes related to the measured concept and then collect data to determine if the results align with these predictions. In a research project evaluating a new depression scale, researchers hypothesized that scores on the scale would inversely correlate with measures of psychological well-being, supporting the construct validity of the instrument. After administering both the new depression scale and established measures of psychological well-being to participants, they found consistently negative correlations, confirming the construct validity of the new scale.

Convergent validity is assessed when researchers employ multiple instruments to measure the same theoretical construct. Convergent validity examines the degree of agreement among observed scores obtained from different assessment tools measuring the same theoretical construct. For example, a study investigating depression, researchers compared scores from two different depression assessment scales, finding a strong positive correlation between them. This correlation supported the convergent validity of both instruments, indicating their ability to measure the same underlying construct effectively.

Conversely, *divergent validity* testing involves comparing scores from instruments measuring distinct theoretical constructs, often contrasting opposing concepts like depression and happiness, were negative correlations support construct validity. The integration of convergent and divergent testing forms a strategy known as multitrait-multimethod, particularly effective in mitigating systematic error.

The *known group* approach is another method used to assess construct validity. In this approach, instruments are administered to individuals who are categorized as either high or low on the characteristic being measured. Researchers anticipate significant score differences between the high and low groups. As an example of the known group approach, researchers may administer an anxiety assessment to individuals known to have diagnosed anxiety disorders and compare their scores with those of individuals without such disorders. If the assessment accurately distinguishes between the two groups, it demonstrates construct validity.

Furthermore, constructs often encompass multiple dimensions, known as factors. To identify these factors, researchers employ *factor analysis*, a statistical technique that groups questions based on their correlations. Items that cluster together strongly indicate high correlations within the same factor, while those that do not align may be revised or removed. Given the intricate computations involved in factor analysis, computers are indispensable for conducting this analysis effectively.

2.6.3 Reliability

Reliability pertains to the consistency of measurements obtained over time, which must be considered in conjunction with validity. While an instrument can be reliable, it may lack validity. For example, if a nurse consistently uses the same pain assessment tool for patients and obtains similar pain scores each time, it indicates the reliability of the tool in measuring pain intensity. However, if the nurse were to use the pain assessment tool to assess other factors like anxiety or depression, its reliability in measuring pain would not necessarily imply validity in assessing those psychological states.

Reliability estimates are often expressed as correlation coefficients, typically ranging from 0.00 to +1.00. Coefficients above 0.80 are deemed acceptable for established instruments, while those exceeding 0.70 are acceptable for newly developed ones. This distinction is crucial as it reflects the nature of relationships tested within the reliability framework. The evaluation of instrument reliability focuses on three key attributes: *stability*, *equivalence*, and *internal consistency* [21]. Stability pertains to the consistency of scores obtained through repeated measurements under identical conditions, exemplified by the analogy of the pain assessment scale. Equivalence is attained when different forms of the instrument or assessments by various raters yield consistent results. Internal consistency, also known as homogeneity, is evident when all items within a questionnaire measure the same underlying concept. Researchers commonly employ seven methods to assess instrument reliability, which include test-retest reliability, parallel or alternate form reliability, inter-rater reliability, split-half reliability, item-total correlation, the Kuder–Richardson coefficient, and Cronbach's alpha.

2.6.3.1 Stability
Test-retest reliability assesses stability by administering the instrument to the same group of subjects under identical conditions on two separate occasions. This method utilizes Pearson's correlation coefficient (r) to calculate the degree of consistency between the scores obtained at the two time points. On the other hand, parallel or alternate form testing evaluates both stability and equivalence by presenting participants with different versions of the instrument. These versions, known as *parallel forms*, feature alterations in wording or layout while maintaining similarity in content. Consequently, researchers anticipate strong positive correlations between scores from the different forms. For instance, when administering an anxiety assessment to individuals diagnosed with anxiety disorders, consistent scores across different forms would support the reliability and equivalence of the instrument.

2.6.3.2 Equivalence
Equivalence is assessed through *inter-rater reliability*, which involves qualitatively evaluating the agreement between two or more observers. One approach to evaluating inter-rater reliability involves having two observers independently score the same event, followed by a comparison

of their ratings. Consistency between the ratings indicates robust reliability of the instrument.

For example, in clinical settings, inter-rater reliability might be evaluated when multiple nurses independently assess a patient's pain level using a pain scale. The level of agreement among the nurses' assessments reflects the inter-rater reliability of the pain scale. If all nurses consistently assign similar scores to the patient's pain level, it suggests high inter-rater reliability of the pain scale in capturing the patient's subjective experience of pain. In research contexts, researchers might assign scores to items on an instrument based on their relevance. The consistency among their scores indicates the instrument's inter-rater reliability.

2.6.3.3 Internal Consistency
Internal consistency reliability assesses whether different test items addressing the same concept produce similar outcomes. This evaluation ensures the uniformity of items within a scale or measure. Unlike other reliability measures that necessitate repeated testing, it can be determined in a single testing session, reducing associated challenges. Typically, it is represented in two primary formats: inter-item consistency and split-half reliability.

Inter-item consistency refers to the degree of uniformity in collecting information, ensuring that data are gathered consistently across various items within a measurement instrument. It confirms the comparability of responses obtained from different items intended to measure the same construct. This reliability measure is vital because variations in how respondents interpret different items may lead to discrepancies in assessing the knowledge or skills demonstrated.

For example, in clinical nursing practice, inter-item consistency could be examined when developing a patient assessment tool for assessing pain management effectiveness. Suppose the assessment tool includes items related to pain intensity, pain location, and pain relief interventions. Nurses would use these items to evaluate a patient's pain experience and the effectiveness of interventions. Inter-item consistency would be assessed by analyzing whether responses to items within each category (pain intensity, location, interventions) are consistently correlated. A high level of inter-item consistency would indicate that all items within each category effectively measure different aspects of pain management, providing nurses with reliable information to guide patient care decisions.

The most common measure of internal consistency is Cronbach's alpha (α), interpreted as the mean of all possible split-half coefficients. It varies between 0 and 1, with 0 indicating no relationship among the items on a scale, and 1 indicating absolute internal consistency. Alpha values above 0.7 are generally acceptable and satisfactory, those above 0.8 are considered quite good, and those above 0.9 reflect exceptional internal consistency. The acceptable range of alpha value estimates is from 0.7 to 0.8. In cases where the level of measurement is dichotomous, internal consistency is assessed using the Kuder-Richardson coefficient (K-20), which evaluates all items simultaneously.

Split-half reliability is a method used to assess the internal consistency of a measurement instrument by comparing the scores of one half of the items with the scores of the other half. The process typically involves administering the entire test to a group of individuals and then dividing the test into two equal halves. If the two halves of the test yield similar scores, it suggests that the test has internal reliability. However, if there are significant discrepancies between the scores of the two halves, it may indicate inconsistency or lack of reliability in the measurement instrument.

This method offers a quick and easy way to establish reliability, but it is only effective with large questionnaires in which all questions measure the same construct. Therefore, it may not be suitable for tests that assess multiple constructs or dimensions. Overall, split-half reliability offers a valuable tool for assessing the internal consistency of measurement instruments, particularly in situations where administering lengthy tests repeatedly may not be feasible.

In reviewing the methods section of research articles, nurses must prioritize the assessment of validity and reliability to inform practice decisions effectively. It is essential that the report includes comprehensive information regarding the validity and reliability of all instruments utilized, along with references to their original development. Some researchers even include the instruments within their articles, facilitating readers to observe how the questions correspond to the measured concepts.

References

1. Grove SK, Gray JR. Understanding nursing research: building an evidence-based practice. Amsterdam: Elsevier; 2022.
2. Pyo J, Lee W, Choi EY, et al. Qualitative research in healthcare: necessity and characteristics. J Prev Med Public Health. 2023;56:12–20. https://doi.org/10.3961/jpmph.22.451.
3. Schmidt NA, Brown JM. Evidence-based practice for nurses: appraisal and application of research. 4th ed. Burlington: Jones & Bartlett Learning; 2024.
4. Fischer HE, Boone WJ, Neumann K. Quantitative research designs and approaches. In: Handbook of research on science education. Milton Park: Routledge; 2023.
5. Houser J. Nursing research: reading, using, and creating evidence. 5th ed. Burlington: Jones & Bartlett Learning; 2023.
6. Kerlinger FN. Foundations of behavioral research. 2nd ed. Hounslow: Surjeet; 2004.
7. Campbell DT, Stanley JC. Experimental and quasi-experimental designs for research. Boston: Ravenio Books; 2015.
8. Melnyk BM, Fineout-Overholt E. Evidence-based practice in nursing & healthcare: a guide to best practice. 5th North American ed. Philadelphia: LWW; 2023.
9. Reichardt CS. Quasi-experimentation: a guide to design and analysis. New York: Guilford; 2019.
10. Lohr SL. Sampling: design and analysis. 3rd ed. New York: Chapman and Hall/CRC; 2021.
11. Stevens SS. On the theory of scales of measurement. Science. 1946;103:677–80. https://doi.org/10.1126/science.103.2684.677.
12. Grove SK, Cipher DJ. Statistics for nursing research: a workbook for evidence-based practice. 4th ed. Amsterdam: Elsevier; 2024.
13. Godshall M. Fast facts for evidence-based practice in nursing. Berlin: Springer; 2024.

14. Polit D, Beck C. Essentials of nursing research: appraising evidence for nursing practice. 10th ed. Philadelphia: LWW; 2021.
15. Mathai AM, Provost SB, Haubold HJ. Multivariate statistical analysis in the real and complex domains. Berlin: Springer; 2023.
16. Hayes AF. Introduction to Mediation, Moderation, and Conditional Process Analysis: A Regression-Based Approach. New York: Guilford Publications; 2022.
17. Zhao Y, Chen (Din) Ding-Geng. Modern Statistical Methods for Health Research. Switzerland: Springer International Publishing; 2022.
18. Bekker A, Ferreira JT, Arashi M, Chen D-G. Innovations in multivariate statistical modeling: navigating theoretical and multidisciplinary domains. Berlin: Springer; 2023.
19. Tappen RM. Advanced nursing research: from theory to practice: from theory to practice. 3rd ed. Burlington: Jones & Bartlett Learning; 2022.
20. Cooper C. An introduction to psychometrics and psychological assessment: using, interpreting and developing tests. New York: Routledge, Chapman & Hall, Incorporated; 2023.
21. Lovett BJ. Practical psychometrics a guide for test users. New York: Guilford; 2023.

Qualitative Nursing Research

3

1. Understand the foundational principles and methodologies of qualitative research in nursing.
2. Differentiate between various qualitative research approaches, such as phenomenology, grounded theory, and ethnography.
3. Apply appropriate qualitative data collection methods, including interviews, focus groups, and observations.
4. Address ethical considerations and challenges in conducting qualitative research in healthcare settings.
5. Conduct qualitative data analysis using coding and thematic analysis techniques.
6. Integrate qualitative research findings into nursing practice to improve patient-centered care.

3.1 Introduction

Qualitative research is a systematic method designed to capture and describe experiences and situations from the viewpoints of the individuals involved. This approach involves the researcher interpreting participants' words to uncover meanings and provide a detailed portrayal of their experiences, fostering a deeper understanding. In nursing, where core values include caring for people and a desire to assist them, qualitative research offers valuable insights into patients' and families' lives. These rich descriptions enhance nurses' comprehension of effective intervention and support strategies, ultimately improving patient care. By embracing qualitative research, nurses can better understand and address the unique needs and circumstances of their patients.

In the field of nursing research, qualitative methodologies play a crucial role in providing in-depth insights and fostering a deeper understanding of patient experiences and healthcare practices. Nurses and healthcare professionals often employ qualitative research to explore the nuanced aspects of patient care, the emotional and psychological outcomes of treatments, and the complexities of healthcare interactions. This chapter aims to elucidate the foundational principles that underpin qualitative research in the context of nursing, emphasizing its significance in enhancing empathetic and holistic care.

A defining characteristic of qualitative research is its commitment to capturing the richness of human experiences through the use of flexible and adaptive methods. Researchers design studies that prioritize the voices of participants, ensuring that data collection techniques such as interviews, focus groups, and observations are sensitive and responsive to the context. Through the lens of qualitative inquiry, this chapter will delve into the intricacies of designing and implementing studies in nursing research,

© The Author(s), under exclusive license to Springer Nature Switzerland AG 2024
M. Al Maqbali, *Essential Research for Evidence-Based Practice in Nursing Care*,
https://doi.org/10.1007/978-3-031-78298-5_3

addressing the unique challenges and ethical considerations inherent in exploring personal and sensitive health-related experiences. By embracing qualitative research, nursing professionals can gain profound insights that contribute to more personalized and compassionate patient care.

Additionally, this chapter will explore the interpretive analyses integral to qualitative research, unraveling the complexities of understanding narrative data in the context of nursing studies. Mastering qualitative methods is essential for researchers and practitioners alike, as it enables them to derive meaningful insights from participants' experiences and make informed decisions that enhance patient care and healthcare policies.

Overall, this chapter serves as a comprehensive guide for nursing researchers seeking to engage with qualitative methodologies. By navigating through the fundamental concepts, methodologies, and interpretive analyses, readers will gain a nuanced understanding of how qualitative research contributes to the advancement of nursing knowledge and practice.

Qualitative research methods involve the systematic investigation of social phenomena through the collection, analysis, and interpretation of textual or visual data. The primary aim of qualitative research is to explore variables and uncover deeper meanings, allowing researchers to draw interpretive conclusions and gain a rich understanding of a population or phenomenon. This approach relies on flexible research designs, adaptive data collection techniques, and thematic analysis to examine patterns, themes, and narratives in data. The overarching goal of qualitative research is to provide a comprehensive and interpretive understanding of the studied phenomena, addressing questions related to "why," "how," or "in what context," and thereby contributing valuable insights to the broader body of knowledge.

In contrast to quantitative research, qualitative research emphasizes understanding and interpreting phenomena or events through words rather than numbers. It focuses on capturing rich, detailed narratives by telling stories, describing events, analyzing case studies, and examining contexts, prioritizing textual over numerical data. While quantitative research aims to draw conclusions through deduction and hypothesis testing, qualitative research is more exploratory and inductive, seeking to uncover deeper meanings and insights. This approach allows researchers to delve into the complexities of human experiences, providing a nuanced understanding that complements the statistical focus of quantitative methods.

3.2 Design

In disciplines such as education, sociology, psychology, and healthcare in general, researchers, students, and practitioners are actively engaging in qualitative studies. Each discipline poses different questions and uses distinct strategies, reflecting the diversity within qualitative research. Authors of qualitative texts have categorized these varied approaches in multiple ways, demonstrating the flexibility and broad applicability of qualitative methods across different domains.

Patton [1] identifies 16 "theoretical traditions" in qualitative research, ranging from well-known classifications like ethnography and grounded theory to less common ones such as semiotics and chaos theory. Denzin et al. [2] contribute to this diversity by discussing several major "strategies of inquiry," including case study, ethnography, grounded theory, and participatory action research. Tesch [3] offers a more extensive list of 45 approaches, categorized into designs, data analysis techniques, and disciplinary orientations. Creswell and Poth [4] simplify this into five main "approaches": narrative research, phenomenology, grounded theory, ethnography, and case study. This overview illustrates the lack of consensus on classifying the myriad approaches to qualitative research, highlighting the complexity and variety of methods available.

In nursing, given the variety of qualitative research strategies, five of the more commonly used approaches to conducting qualitative research are presented. These methodologies have been encountered throughout many years of experience advising doctoral students, teaching qualitative research courses, and conducting qualitative research: basic qualitative research, phenomenology, grounded theory, ethnography, historical, and qualitative case study.

Although these methodologies are typically grouped under the qualitative research umbrella, they each provide unique perspectives and methodologies that impact various aspects, including formulating research questions, selecting samples, collecting and analyzing data, and presenting findings. Moreover, researchers have the flexibility to combine multiple methodologies, such as incorporating ethnography into a case study, to offer a holistic understanding of nursing phenomena.

3.2.1   Phenomenology

Phenomenology forms the foundation of qualitative research, leading to the common misconception that all qualitative research is inherently phenomenological. Phenomenology refers to both a philosophy and a set of research methods aligned with that philosophy, focusing on the study of experiences or phenomena [5]. The philosophy of phenomenology emphasizes the essence of experiences and the process through which these experiences become part of our consciousness. Unlike modern science, which aims to categorize, simplify, and reduce phenomena to abstract principles, phenomenologists focus on **lived experiences** [6]. This approach requires direct engagement with phenomena, which are often obscured by theoretical frameworks [7].

Essentially, phenomenology examines people's conscious experiences of their everyday life and social interactions, with the broad research question being, "What is this lived experience like?" [8]. In phenomenological research, data is collected from individuals who have experienced the phenomenon under study, aiming to distil a composite essence of that experience [4]. Phenomenologists hold diverse philosophical views, with nursing researchers often grounding their study designs in the works of early phenomenologists like Husserl [5] or Heidegger [9].

3.2.1.1 Descriptive Phenomenology

Descriptive phenomenology, established by Husserl, focuses strictly on the phenomena themselves, striving to capture the essence of experience without any interpretation, explanation, or theorizing [5]. Through the analysis of meaning-laden statements, researchers can uncover the inherent structure within the phenomenon. Husserl's philosophy underpins descriptive phenomenological research, which seeks to describe experiences as they are lived, or in phenomenological terms, to capture the "lived experience" of study participants. To accurately describe lived experiences, Husserl posits that researchers must bracket or set aside their biases and preconceptions, allowing them to describe the phenomenon in a naïve, unbiased manner [10]. This method provides a foundational approach to understanding the core of human experiences in their purest form.

3.2.1.2 Interpretive Phenomenology (Hermeneutics)

Interpretive phenomenology, or hermeneutic phenomenology, focuses on interpreting and comprehending the meanings of experiences within their specific contexts. This method involves a dialogical process between the researcher and participants, where the researcher's interpretations and reflections are crucial in uncovering deeper meanings. Interpretive phenomenology seeks to explore how individuals make sense of their experiences and how these experiences are embedded within broader social, cultural, and historical contexts.

Heidegger argued that it is impossible to set aside one's preconceptions and understand the world naively. He believed phenomenological researchers should describe how participants interpret their experiences, then analyze these interpretations for hidden meanings. Interpretive phenomenological research, following Heidegger's philosophy, involves presenting a rich, interpretive description of phenomena. For example, in patient care, hermeneutics can help nurse researchers understand how patients interpret their diagnoses and how these interpretations affect their roles in critical issues in nursing research and practice, such as life, death, and pain. This approach enables the interpretation of phenomena to provide a clearer understanding of what the nurse researcher intends to convey, emphasizing the psychological implications of language or specific words in context.

3.2.2 Grounded Theory

Grounded theory, developed by Glaser and Strauss in 1967, originated from real-life observations of how individuals approach the process of dying [11]. This approach derives theories from data that are systematically gathered and analyzed throughout the research process. Instead of testing pre-existing theories empirically, grounded theory emphasizes **developing** new theories that are rooted directly in the data. In this method, data collection and analysis occur first, leading to the emergence of a theory that is inherently grounded in the collected data.

Grounded theory differs from other qualitative research methods through its emphasis on theory construction. Nurses found the method appealing due to its relevance to the life experiences of individuals dealing with health issues and its capacity to create interpretations of human behavior [12]. In nursing research, a grounded theory study might explore how new nurses adapt to their first year of practice. By systematically collecting and analyzing data from real-life observations and interviews, researchers could develop a theory about the stages of adaptation and effective coping strategies [13]. This theory, grounded in the nurses' actual experiences, would provide specific insights to inform training programs and support systems, aiding new nurses in their transition. These theories are detailed and practical, making them especially valuable for real-world application, unlike more generalized theories [14]. Moreover, grounded theory is particularly effective for investigating processes, such as how something evolves over time.

The grounded theory method employs both inductive and deductive strategies in developing theories [15]. Constructs and concepts are rooted in the data, and hypotheses are examined as they emerge from the research process. There is a contention that, considering the current stage of nursing theory development, generating theories holds greater significance than testing them for the progression of nursing knowledge. This approach allows for the emergence of new insights and a deeper understanding of complex phenomena within the nursing field, ultimately contributing to more effective and tailored nursing practices.

3.2.3 Ethnography

Ethnographic research, initially devised by anthropologists, involves immersing oneself in a **culture** to understand how it evolves and sustains itself over time. This method allows researchers to study a community with a shared culture, examining their origins, historical lifestyles, and survival strategies. Ethnography also refers to the written account resulting from such studies. Early ethnographers often focused on examining cultures that were considered primitive, foreign, or remote. Today, ethnographic methods are also applied to modern and urban cultures, providing valuable insights into contemporary social dynamics.

The philosophical foundation of ethnographic research lies in anthropology, acknowledging that culture encompasses both material and nonmaterial elements. Material culture includes all tangible creations and constructions, such as buildings for cultural events, cultural symbols, family traditions, social networks, and beliefs manifested in social and political institutions. Nonmaterial culture, consisting of symbolic meanings, social customs, and beliefs, may only become evident over time within a different culture but are crucial to understanding it. Cultures also possess ideals that are considered desirable, even if people do not always adhere to them. Anthropologists and nurse ethnographers aim to uncover the various components of a culture and understand their interconnections, gradually forming a comprehensive picture of the culture as a whole.

Ethnoscience is an anthropological method employed to uncover nursing knowledge. Ethnonursing involves the organized study and classification of nursing care beliefs, values, and practices within a specific culture [16]. Cultural members convey their insights on nursing phenomena, such as care, health, and the environment, through their language, experiences, beliefs, and value systems. Since ethnonursing focuses specifically on nursing, the scope and depth of these studies are typically narrower than those aimed at understanding an entire culture. Consequently, gathering information may not necessitate prolonged immersion in the culture.

The ethnographic researcher must deeply acquaint themselves with the culture under study by observing, actively participating, and interviewing its members. Even in focused ethnographies, immersion in the culture is essential. This immersion involves spending significant time within the culture and gaining a deep understanding of its various aspects, such as language, sociocultural norms, traditions, and other social dimensions, including family dynamics, communication patterns (both verbal and nonverbal), religious practices, work routines, and emotional expressions [4]. Through this process, the researcher becomes increasingly accepted by the community.

While ethnographic researchers need to be actively involved in the culture they are studying, they must maintain a critical distance to avoid "going native," a situation where they become so integrated into the culture that they lose their objectivity and ability to observe clearly [4]. Maintaining this balance ensures the integrity and accuracy of data collection and analysis. Additionally, researchers often document their experiences and reflections in field notes, which serve as valuable resources for understanding and interpreting cultural phenomena.

3.2.4 Historical

Historical research involves the systematic collection, critical evaluation, and interpretation of historical evidence, which includes data related to **past** events [1]. This type of research aims to answer questions about the causes, effects, or trends of historical occurrences to gain insights into present behaviors or practices. Understanding contemporary nursing theories, practices, or issues can often be enriched by investigating specific segments of the past. For instance, many nurse researchers have conducted biographical studies focusing on the experiences or contributions of notable individuals, such as nursing leaders.

Additionally, other researchers have examined the development and impact of significant nursing movements or organizations, such as the establishment of the first nursing schools or the role of nursing associations in advancing the profession. This approach not only preserves the legacy of influential figures but also provides valuable lessons and perspectives that can inform current nursing practice and education. Additionally, historical research helps in identifying long-term trends and shifts in nursing, contributing to a deeper understanding of the profession's evolution.

Currently, some historians are focusing on the lives and experiences of everyday people, often investigating topics such as social roles, ethnic backgrounds, and socioeconomic status. Other researchers focus on social histories, exploring particular periods to understand the prevailing values and beliefs that influenced subsequent developments [4]. Moreover, some historians engage in intellectual histories, analyzing historical ideas or ways of thinking. This broadened focus in historical research provides a more comprehensive understanding of the diverse forces that have shaped societies over time.

Historical research should not be mistaken for a mere review of literature on historical events. Unlike literature reviews, which summarize existing knowledge, historical inquiry aims to discover new insights. One significant difference is that historical researchers are frequently motivated by specific hypotheses, questions, or theoretical perspectives, which may include various ideological frameworks [14]. These hypotheses in historical research seek to explain and interpret the conditions, events, or phenomena being studied. Instead of being tested statistically, they are generally stated as broad conjectures about the relationships among historical events, trends, and phenomena [17]. This approach allows researchers to delve deeper into the complexities of history, uncovering connections and patterns that contribute to our understanding of the past.

3.2.5 Case Studies

Case studies are thorough examinations of individuals or groups, and they can also focus on institutions, such as hospice care for the terminally ill. Originating in sociology, the case study method has been extensively utilized in anthropology, law, and medicine. In medicine, case studies often focus on specific diseases. In nursing, case studies involve in-depth investigations of a single entity or a small number of entities, which could be an individual, a family, an institution, or another social unit. Case study researchers strive to understand issues that are significant to the context of the focal entity. Additionally, case studies provide valuable insights into complex real-world situations, offering a detailed and nuanced understanding of the subject matter.

A case study involves the **in-depth** analysis and detailed description of various subjects, such as an individual's activities, special needs, life circumstances, and personal history [18]. It can also focus on groups of people, like a school department or teaching staff as well as specific problems, processes, phenomena, or events within a particular institution. For example, in nursing, a case study might examine the teamwork and communication practices within a hospital's ICU staff or the impact of a new patient care protocol on nurse performance and patient outcomes. If the analysis remains purely descriptive, the case study is classified as a descriptive method. However, if the analysis explores cause-and-effect relationships, the case study advances toward a causal experimental method [19]. By incorporating both descriptive and causal analyses, case studies can provide a comprehensive understanding of complex situations.

The term "case study" is well-known in the nursing profession as a teaching tool used to analyze a patient's clinical case. However, case study research is less commonly employed and is similarly defined by methodologists as a research approach that focuses on a single phenomenon, variable, or set of variables occurring within a specific context of time and place. This approach aims to gain a comprehensive understanding of the phenomenon under investigation.

The subject of a case study can be an individual, group, organization, or event. The primary objective of case study research is to explore the "how" or "why" a phenomenon functions, in contrast to other qualitative research methods that aim to define the "what" of a phenomenon. Conducting case study research typically involves a detailed examination over an extended period, capturing present and past experiences, situational factors, and relevant interrelationships. While some authors classify case study research strictly as a qualitative methodology, others view it as flexible, incorporating both qualitative and quantitative evidence. Additionally, this approach is particularly valuable for uncovering deep insights into complex issues within real-world contexts.

3.3   Theoretical Frameworks

In nursing research, qualitative methods are grounded in the belief that there is no single, observable reality. Researchers employing these methods develop their findings inductively, progressing from raw data to a comprehensive conceptual understanding. Theoretical frameworks can be instrumental in guiding qualitative analyses by highlighting relevant concepts and relationships to explore [20, 21]. These frameworks can help shape the narrative that emerges from the analysis. At the same time, the rich, detailed descriptions provided by the analysis can deepen the understanding and appreciation of the theoretical framework. However, it is important to be mindful that the use of a theoretical framework might limit inductive reasoning or lead to conclusions that do not align with the data [22]. Therefore, nurses must strike a balance between utilizing theoretical frameworks and maintaining an open, unbiased approach to data interpretation. This balanced approach ensures that the findings remain true to the experiences and realities of the patients and phenomena being studied.

A theoretical framework can be highly useful in qualitative nursing research. It describes concepts and relationships within a given phenomenon, effectively serving as a map for qualitative exploration [4]. These frameworks may be developed inductively from previous research or derived from existing theories and literature. A theoretical framework is particularly beneficial when there is an abundance of data, as it helps direct the researcher's attention to specific phenomena of interest [23]. This focused approach facilitates a deeper and more organized analysis, ensuring that the research remains relevant and meaningful within the context of nursing practice.

A theoretical framework can enhance qualitative nursing research by providing a sense of the emerging narrative from the analyses, guiding inquiries that might otherwise be overlooked [1, 15]. It can transform a simple question about a phenomenon into a comprehensive investigation. The framework offers an orientation, while rigorous data analysis yields insightful findings. Additionally, the rich descriptions from the analysis can lead to a deeper appreciation of the theoretical framework. The framework becomes more refined through its alignment with the data, and the data are understood from a fresh perspective [18]. However, employing a theoretical framework in qualitative inquiry carries the risk of biasing findings or constraining inductive discovery [24]. Thus, the goal is to maximize the utility of a theoretical framework without forcing the data to fit into a preconceived structure, ensuring that the findings remain authentic and true to the nursing context.

3.4   Sampling

Qualitative research aims to gain insights and uncover meanings related to specific phenomena, situations, events, or cultural elements. It typically utilizes small, nonrandom samples that are deliberately chosen to provide detailed and in-depth insights. The objective is to develop a deep understanding from a carefully selected group, rather than to generalize the findings to a larger population, as is the case in quantitative research. In qualitative studies, the focus of sampling is more on experiences, events, incidents, and settings rather than on individuals.

The samples are selected based on specific characteristics or criteria relevant to the research question, rather than aiming for statistical representativeness. This approach allows researchers to explore complex phenomena, understand diverse perspectives, and gather rich, contextual data that might be missed with larger, random samples. For some studies, recruiting participants with diverse characteristics (heterogeneous sampling) provides a broader range of experiences. This approach is often used in grounded theory studies to support the development of a comprehensive theory. In other studies, participants may share similar characteristics (homogeneous sampling), particularly when the central focus is on a specific phenomenon. This ensures a deeper understanding of the phenomenon within a specific context. It is essential to choose the sampling method that best aligns with the research objectives to obtain meaningful and relevant data.

In qualitative research, individuals are referred to as participants because the researcher and participants collaboratively conduct the study. Sampling in qualitative research is intentional and purposeful, with participants selected for their specific knowledge, experience, or perspectives relevant to the study. Researchers may also employ additional sampling methods, such as network and theoretical sampling, depending on the study's focus. For example, in ethnographic studies, researchers often first choose the setting and site, followed by the population and phenomenon of interest. This method allows for a rich, contextual exploration of the research topic, providing nuanced insights that might be overlooked with other sampling approaches. Additionally, this focused approach ensures that the data collected is highly relevant and specific to the research questions being addressed.

In phenomenological research, researchers typically begin by selecting the phenomenon or population of interest and then identify potential participants for their studies. These participants must have relevant experience and knowledge in the area of study and be willing to provide rich, in-depth information about the phenomenon, situation, culture, or event being examined. For instance, if the study aims to explore the experience of caring for a loved one with dementia, the researcher will select individuals who are articulate and reflective, have substantial caregiving experience, and are willing to share their caregiving journey. Additionally, the participants should be able to offer detailed personal insights that can contribute to a deeper understanding of the phenomenon under investigation.

3.4.1   Types of Qualitative Samples

Qualitative researchers generally steer clear of probability samples, as random sampling is not suitable for selecting individuals who make effective informants—those who are knowledgeable, articulate, reflective, and willing to participate in in-depth discussions. Instead, they use various nonprobability sampling methods, which allow for the selection of participants capable of providing rich, insightful data. The chosen sampling strategy is vital for ensuring the study's depth and relevance, directly influencing the quality and richness of the information collected.

Common sampling methods in qualitative nursing research include purposeful sampling, network or snowball sampling, theoretical sampling, and convenience sampling. Because the sample selection process profoundly affects the study's quality, researchers must describe their sampling methods in detail to facilitate proper interpretation of the findings. This detailed description helps ensure the study's credibility and enables others to understand the context and rationale behind the participant selection.

3.4.1.1 Convenience Sampling
Convenience sampling, also known as volunteer sampling in qualitative research, is occasionally employed when researchers require potential participants to step forward and self-identify. For example, when studying the experiences of individuals dealing with chronic insomnia, it can be difficult to swiftly gather a sizable participant pool. In such scenarios, recruitment strategies might entail distributing flyers in community centers, advertising in health-related magazines, or utilizing online forums to attract individuals experiencing chronic sleep difficulties. While this method may not ensure a fully representative sample, it emphasizes the assembly of a diverse cohort encompassing various aspects of the insomnia experience.

Although convenience sampling may offer ease and efficiency, it is generally not the preferred method, even in qualitative studies. The primary aim in qualitative research is to extract the most informative insights from the sample, and convenience sampling may not always yield the most information-rich sources. However, it can serve as a cost-effective and straightforward starting point for the sampling process, with other methods potentially employed as data collection progresses.

3.4.1.2 Purposeful Sampling
Purposeful sampling, also known as judgmental or selective sampling, involves the deliberate selection of specific participants, elements, events, or incidents for inclusion in a study. Researchers may intentionally include both typical and atypical participants, or similar and varied situations, to enrich the understanding of the phenomenon under investigation. For instance, in a study examining the experiences of caregivers for Alzheimer's patients, researchers might include caregivers who have been providing care for different durations and who care for patients at various stages of the disease to capture a wide range of perspectives. The primary objective of purposeful sampling is to select cases that offer rich and detailed information for the study.

Critics of purposeful sampling argue that it may be challenging to evaluate the accuracy or relevance of the researcher's judgment. To address this concern, researchers should transparently report the desired characteristics of study participants and provide a rationale for their selection, ensuring the collection of essential data. In qualitative research, purposeful sampling is often considered the most effective approach for gaining insights into new areas of study, uncovering new meanings, and achieving a comprehensive understanding of complex experiences, situations, or events. Additionally, this sampling method allows researchers to focus on specific aspects of the phenomenon of interest, leading to deeper insights and richer data.

3.4.1.3 Snowball Sampling

In qualitative research, snowball sampling involves asking initial informants to refer other potential study participants. Also known as nominated or network sampling, this method relies on the recommendations of those already included in the sample. This approach is particularly useful for accessing individuals who are difficult to identify through other means.

Snowball sampling offers several advantages over convenience sampling. First, it can be more cost-efficient and practical, reducing the time researchers spend screening individuals to determine their suitability for the study. Additionally, being introduced by a referring participant can help researchers establish trust more easily with new participants. This method also allows researchers to specify desired characteristics in new participants more readily. For instance, in a study exploring the experiences of nurses working in high-stress clinical environments, researchers could ask initial participants if they know other nurses who work in similar settings and are willing to share their experiences. This approach would help researchers gather insights from a broader range of clinical nursing professionals, enhancing the depth and richness of the study.

However, this approach has some limitations. The final sample might be confined to a narrow network of acquaintances, potentially limiting the diversity of perspectives. Furthermore, the quality of referrals may depend on whether the initial participants trust the researcher and are genuinely willing to cooperate. To mitigate these weaknesses, researchers should carefully manage the referral process and strive to ensure a broad and varied sample. Additionally, combining snowball sampling with other methods can help enhance the overall robustness and diversity of the participant pool.

3.4.1.4 Theoretical Sampling

Theoretical sampling is a strategy in qualitative research aimed at developing a specific theory or model throughout the research process. This approach is particularly common in grounded theory research. Researchers using theoretical sampling gather data from individuals or groups who can provide diverse, rich, and relevant information critical for theory development. The data are considered valuable if they contribute to the generation, delimitation, and saturation of theoretical codes necessary for the study. A code is deemed saturated when it is fully understood, and its role in the theory is clear. If any code or concept remains ambiguous, the researcher continues to seek additional participants and collect more data. This iterative process persists until all codes are saturated, leading to the emergence of the theory from the collected data and codes. The course of theoretical sampling is guided by the evolving grounded theory, which directs researchers through various directions and lines of inquiry, rather than following a linear path.

It is important to distinguish theoretical sampling from purposive sampling. While purposive sampling focuses on selecting participants based on predetermined criteria, theoretical sampling aims to uncover categories and their properties, as well as to reveal the interrelationships within the substantive theory. The fundamental question guiding theoretical sampling is: "Which groups or subgroups should be explored next in data collection?" These groups are not preselected but are chosen as needed during the research process to contribute to the development of emerging categories.

Diversity within the sample is highly encouraged to ensure that the developed theory encompasses a broad range of behaviors across various situations and settings. This diversity strengthens the robustness and applicability of the theory. For example, in a study aimed at understanding the stress management strategies employed by nurses, the researcher would seek out nurses from various units such as intensive care, surgical, and mental health. This approach ensures the theory captures a comprehensive range of stress management techniques used in different clinical settings within the nursing profession.

3.4.2   Sample Size in Qualitative Research

There are no strict criteria or rules for determining sample size in qualitative research. Instead, it primarily depends on the study's objectives, the quality of the participants, and the chosen sampling strategy. The final number of participants, sites, and artifacts is determined by the depth of information required to understand a phenomenon, describe a cultural element, develop a theory, or explain a significant healthcare concept or issue. Researchers may continue to recruit additional participants during data collection and analysis to ensure high-quality findings. It is a common misconception that the number of samples is irrelevant to the adequacy of the sampling strategy. In reality, the effectiveness and strength of various purposeful sampling methods in qualitative research depend primarily on the richness and quality of information obtained from each sampling unit, rather than the number of units sampled. Therefore, a key principle is **data saturation** continuing to sample until no new information emerges and redundancy is achieved.

Saturation originates from grounded theory, introduced by Glaser and Strauss, as a method for creating theoretical and interpretive frameworks from qualitative data. Glaser and Strauss [11] defined saturation as the criterion for deciding when to stop sampling—this point is reached when no new data emerge that develop the properties of a category, and similar instances recur repeatedly, allowing the researcher to be empiri-

cally confident that data saturation has been achieved [25]. Essentially, saturation signifies the point at which additional sampling yields no new insights. This concept indicates that sampling and data analysis are interconnected processes that occur concurrently, rather than sequentially. In grounded theory, the concept referred to is theoretical saturation. Theoretical saturation occurs when no further themes or insights surface during data collection, and all conceptual categories have been thoroughly examined, identified, and finalized [26]. This signifies that the data collection process has reached a point where no new significant information is being generated, ensuring comprehensive coverage of the study's focal areas.

This integrated approach ensures that the development of conceptual categories is closely tied to the data being collected and analyzed. Therefore, understanding when to stop sampling is crucial for maintaining the study's rigor and depth.

3.4.3   Sampling in Mean Qualitative Research Design

The sample size is a perennial topic of debate among qualitative researchers. Given that qualitative research typically involves smaller sample sizes, ensuring that the sample is sufficient to achieve data saturation is crucial [25, 27]. While there is no definitive rule for determining sample size in qualitative studies, some researchers suggest that relatively homogeneous populations can reach saturation [28, 29]. Others argue that a larger sample size can enhance the identification of patterns and themes by incorporating a wider range of perspectives and experiences, thereby increasing the likelihood of achieving saturation [30, 31]. However, excessively large qualitative samples can lead to ethical concerns, such as the inefficient use of research funds, undue participant burden, and the unnecessary expenditure of time. Conversely, samples that are too small may fail to reach saturation, undermining the credibility of the study's findings.

3.4.4 Ethnography Sampling

In ethnography, sampling typically involves more than just selecting informants; it also includes observation and other data collection methods, which are crucial for understanding a culture. Ethnographers must decide not only whom to sample but also what to sample. Over the past two decades, methodologists have rigorously examined the concept of saturation. According to a systematic review by [27], achieving saturation often required a narrow range of sample sizes: 9–17 individual interviews or 4–9 focus groups. The qualitative studies reviewed were generally conducted in relatively homogeneous populations with narrow aims. In contrast, studies with broader aims or more diverse populations needed larger sample sizes, ranging from 20 to 40 interviews [27]. This suggests that the required sample size in ethnography is influenced by the homogeneity of the population and the specificity of the research objectives.

Ethnographic research necessitates sampling because it is impossible for the researcher to observe or record every event. The number of participants depends on the diversity within the target population, with the concept of "saturation" indicating when enough data has been collected. Skilled researchers employ multiple methods in the recruitment process and do not adhere strictly to conventional sampling techniques. Instead, ethnography utilizes a nonprobability sample, aimed not at statistical representation but at deliberately selecting individuals to reflect specific characteristics or groups within the population. This approach emphasizes achieving a purposive sample through the use of sample coverage and sample frames, thereby ensuring the research addresses the relevant diversity of the population being studied.

3.4.5 Phenomenological Sampling

Phenomenological research often involves smaller sample sizes compared to other qualitative studies due to the in-depth interaction required between researchers and participants. Formal methods in phenomenological research rarely define adequate sample sizes, with only the interpretative approach providing some guidance. Researchers frequently argue that the quality of phenomenological research is crucial when discussing typical sample sizes and variants in this field [25, 29, 32]. Generally, phenomenological studies involve fewer than ten participants.

A fundamental principle in selecting participants for a phenomenological study is that all individuals must have experienced the phenomenon being investigated and must be able to describe their lived experiences [33]. Thus, phenomenologists typically use a criterion sampling method, where the primary criterion is direct experience with the phenomenon under study. While seeking participants with relevant experiences, phenomenological researchers also aim to capture a diverse range of individual experiences. This diversity enriches the understanding of the phenomenon by highlighting its various facets and nuances.

3.4.6 Grounded Theory Sampling

Grounded theory research typically involves samples of around 20–30 participants, using theoretical sampling [4]. In grounded theory, the objective is to achieve theoretical saturation, which is distinctly different from merely reaching a point where no new data is emerging from fieldwork. Theoretical saturation can only be attained through theoretical sampling, as the goal is to saturate a theoretical construct derived from the data to develop a theoretical account considered the "best fit" for a concept [34]. This process involves researchers choosing a term that best represents the observed pattern of behavior.

Theoretical saturation in data collection is achieved when no new or relevant data emerge regarding a category, the category is thoroughly developed in terms of its properties and dimensions showing variation, and the relationships among categories are well-established and validated [12]. Thus, theoretical saturation ensures a comprehensive understanding of the emerging theory, providing a solid foundation for further research and practical application.

3.5   Data Collection

In qualitative research, data collection is closely tied to sampling and should be seen as complementary. Data are gathered directly from the chosen sample population, ensuring that the information is relevant and specific to the research questions. The collected data can be classified as either 'direct data' or 'indirect data.'

Direct data includes both recorded spoken or written words and observable behaviors, actions, and interactions. These interactions can be between people or reactions to objects. Any observable or communicable element is considered potential or actual data. This includes thoughts, feelings, experiences, meanings of experiences, responses, actions, interactions, language, and processes of individuals and groups within their social and cultural settings. This type of data provides the context for qualitative studies, offering a rich, detailed background for understanding findings.

In a nursing study, direct data might include the recorded verbal responses of patients during interviews, their written feedback on surveys, and the observable interactions between nurses and patients during care. It could also encompass the body language of patients during consultations, the way they respond to different treatments, and their interactions with medical equipment. All these elements create a comprehensive context for the study, allowing researchers to understand the nuances of patient care and the effectiveness of nursing interventions in various social and cultural settings.

Indirect data, on the other hand, is produced by someone or something else initially. This includes documents, photographs capturing an event, or artistic representations of experiences such as novels, songs, paintings, poems, and photographs. In a nursing study, indirect data might include patient medical records, photographs of treatment procedures, or songs and poems written by patients reflecting their healthcare experiences. It could also involve analyzing novels or artworks created by individuals that depict their journeys through illness and recovery. These forms of indirect data provide valuable insights into patients' experiences and the impact of nursing care from a different perspective.

Direct data is the most common form in qualitative research due to its immediacy and depth. Various methods can be used to collect direct data, either individually or in combination, depending on the study's needs. These methods include interviews, observations, open-ended questionnaires, journaling (diary accounts), or "think aloud" sessions. Participants can also be asked by the researcher to collect direct data themselves, such as by keeping a personal journal or diary and then sharing it with the researcher.

Typically, qualitative research gathers data primarily through direct contact with participants, often via interviews, or through the researcher's presence at relevant events, typically through observation. This approach is quite different from quantitative research, which often involves no direct interaction with participants or events.

Additionally, qualitative researchers in nursing must be skilled at navigating the complexities of fieldwork. They need to be flexible and responsive to emerging data, adapting their methods and strategies as needed. This adaptability enables researchers to explore the nuances of patient care and nursing practices, uncovering layers of meaning that might otherwise remain hidden. The ability to creatively solve problems and develop new strategies on the fly is crucial for qualitative researchers, ensuring they can handle unexpected challenges and still gather meaningful, robust data.

The process of qualitative data collection in nursing is dynamic and context-sensitive, requiring a blend of careful planning and adaptive, responsive methods. This combination of structure and flexibility allows qualitative research to provide deep, nuanced insights into patient experiences and nursing practices, enhancing our understanding of healthcare environments and social phenomena within the field.

3.5.1 Interviews

In qualitative research, interviews often serve as a primary method for data collection. An interview can be defined as a process in which the researcher and the participant engage in a structured conversation cantered around questions relevant to the research topic [20]. The most typical interview format involves a one-on-one interaction, where one individual gathers information from another. Alternatively, data can also be collected through group discussions, such as focus groups, where multiple participants share their perspectives on the subject matter. These interviews, whether individual or collective, are crucial for gaining in-depth insights into the participants' experiences, thoughts, and feelings. These interviews can be conducted via telephone or virtual meetings (e.g., Zoom, Microsoft Teams) [35].

The primary goal of an interview is to gather unique insights. The researcher seeks to understand what resides in someone else's mind. The purpose of interviewing is to gain access to another person's perspective, allowing us to see the world through their eyes. Interviews are especially valuable when direct observation of behavior, emotions, or personal interpretations of the surrounding world is not possible [36]. Additionally, interviews are essential when exploring past events that cannot be recreated or directly observed. Through this process, researchers can uncover rich, detailed information that might otherwise remain inaccessible.

Interviewing becomes essential when direct observation of behavior, emotions, or people's interpretations of the world around them is not feasible [1]. It is equally important when the focus is on past events that cannot be recreated or directly witnessed. For example, in nursing research, interviewing patients who have undergone a specific treatment allows the researcher to understand their emotional responses, coping mechanisms, and personal experiences—insights that cannot be fully captured through observation or medical records alone. Through these interviews, researchers can explore the deeper meanings behind patients' actions and thoughts, gaining a richer understanding of their experiences that contributes to improved patient care and outcomes.

3.5.1.1 Types of Interviews

Interviews can be categorized in various ways, depending on their structure and underlying theoretical approach. Three primary types of interviews are distinguished based on the degree of structure involved: structured, semistructured, and unstructured interviews. Additionally, interviews can be shaped by different theoretical perspectives, influencing how questions are framed, and data is interpreted. These approaches can be applied across various formats, including individual interviews, focus groups, and electronic interviews conducted via digital platforms. Each type and format offer unique advantages, allowing researchers to tailor their approach to best suit their research objectives and the context of their study. In qualitative nursing research, interviews can be structured, semistructured and unstructured [14].

In **structured** interviews, also known as standardized interviews, both the questions and their sequence are predetermined. The most structured form of this approach resembles an oral version of a written survey. However, in qualitative research, using a highly structured interview can be problematic. Strictly adhering to a set list of questions may prevent a deep exploration of participants' perspectives and their unique understanding of the world. Instead of revealing genuine insights, this approach might only elicit responses that align with the researcher's preconceived notions. Additionally, such interviews rely on the assumption that all respondents share a common vocabulary and interpret the questions in the same way, which can undermine the depth and richness of the data collected.

Despite these limitations, highly structured interviews can be useful in qualitative research for collecting consistent sociodemographic data, such as participants' age, income, employment history, marital status, and education level. This format is also valuable when the researcher needs all participants to respond to a specific statement or define a particular concept or term. However, to fully capture the complexity of participants' experiences and perspectives, researchers may need to combine structured questions with more flexible, open-ended inquiries that allow for a broader exploration of the subject matter.

The **semistructured** interview occupies a middle ground between structured and unstructured formats. In this type of interview, either all the questions are phrased more flexibly or the interview combines both structured and unstructured questions. Typically, there is a section of the interview designed to gather specific information from all respondents, which is more structured. However, the majority of the interview is guided by a list of topics or questions that are meant to be explored, without predetermined wording or a fixed order. This format gives the researcher the flexibility to adapt to the conversation as it unfolds, allowing them to engage with the respondent's emerging perspective and explore new ideas related to the topic.

The semistructured approach is particularly valuable in qualitative research because it balances the need for consistency with the opportunity to delve deeper into the respondent's unique experiences and viewpoints. By allowing for spontaneity and adaptability, the researcher can uncover richer, more nuanced insights that might be missed in a more rigid interview format. This method is especially useful when the researcher seeks to understand complex behaviors, attitudes, or phenomena that require a more conversational and responsive approach.

The third type of interview is **unstructured** and informal, making it particularly useful when the researcher lacks sufficient knowledge about a phenomenon to ask specific questions. In this approach, there is no predetermined set of questions, and the interview is primarily exploratory. One of the main objectives of an unstructured interview is to gather enough information to formulate more focused questions for later interviews. This method is often used alongside participant observation during the early stages of a qualitative study.

Conducting an unstructured interview requires a skilled researcher, as it demands a high degree of flexibility. While this approach can yield valuable insights and a deeper understanding of the subject, it can also be challenging, as the interviewer may feel overwhelmed by the diversity of viewpoints and the abundance of seemingly unrelated information. As a result, completely unstructured interviewing is rarely the sole method of data collection in qualitative research. Instead, researchers often combine all three types of interviews—structured, semistructured, and unstructured—in a single study. This approach allows for the collection of standardized information, ensures that some open-ended questions are consistently asked of all participants, and provides the opportunity for unstructured exploration, leading to fresh insights and the discovery of new information.

By integrating these different interview formats, researchers can balance the need for consistency with the flexibility to explore complex and evolving phenomena, ultimately enriching the depth and quality of the data collected.

Example:
To illustrate the types of questions you might ask in different interview formats—Structured, semistructured, or unstructured—let us consider how these approaches can be applied to a study on the role of mentoring in the professional development of nurses.

Structured Interview:

In a highly structured interview, you might begin by providing each nurse with a precise definition of mentoring, such as "mentoring is a professional relationship in which an experienced nurse provides guidance and support to a less experienced nurse." After giving this definition, you would ask, "can you identify someone in your nursing career who you consider to be a mentor and explain how they have influenced your professional development?" this ensures that all participants are responding to the same concept, allowing for consistency across interviews and easier comparison of responses.

Semistructured Interview:

In a semistructured interview, the approach would be more flexible. Instead of giving a definition, you could ask, "how do you understand the concept of mentoring in nursing?" or "can you describe a mentoring relationship you've experienced in your nursing career?" this allows nurses to share their personal interpretations of mentoring and describe their experiences in their own words. This format provides some structure to ensure key topics are covered, but also gives the participant room to express their individual perspectives and experiences.

Unstructured Interview:

In an unstructured interview, you would ask very open-ended questions that encourage the nurse to share their story in a more narrative form. For example, you might ask, "can you tell me about your journey in nursing and the people who have influenced you along the way?" or "what factors have been most important in shaping your career as a nurse?" this approach allows the nurse to talk freely about their experiences, potentially revealing unexpected insights or new directions for the research. The unstructured format provides the most flexibility, enabling the researcher to follow the respondent's lead and explore topics in greater depth.

Each approach offers different benefits depending on the research goals. The structured interview ensures consistency and comparability, the semistructured interview allows for both consistency and exploration, and the unstructured interview offers maximum flexibility for deep, qualitative insights. By selecting the appropriate interview format, you can gather the most relevant and meaningful data for your nursing research.

3.5.1.2 Effective Interviewing Techniques

The structure and conduct of interviews are crucial to obtaining high-quality narrative data. Poorly executed interviews can lead to substandard data and overall unsatisfactory results. Mastering the art of conducting interviews involves understanding complex and demanding skills, emphasizing the importance of a structured approach Table 3.1. It is ill-advised to adopt a "learn as you go" method in qualitative research interviews. To ensure preparedness and refine their techniques, researchers often perform practice sessions or "dummy runs" with peers or colleagues, allowing them to pilot and adjust the interview schedule before engaging in actual interviews [37].

Whether novice or experienced, researchers must be properly prepared to conduct interviews within a clinical setting, adhering to certain prerequisites. Early on, it is essential to establish the "rules of engagement," such as consistently exhibiting a warm, non-judgmental demeanor toward participants. This involves asking questions in a balanced, unbiased, non-threatening, sensitive, and clear manner. Moreover, choosing a suitable setting for the interview, especially when addressing personal questions, is crucial for maintaining a comfortable and respectful environment. Most interviews in qualitative research are audio-recorded, with video recording used less frequently. It is vital for researchers to obtain informed consent and explain the recording process to participants to ensure they are comfortable with the method chosen.

During the interview process, it is crucial to prioritize the participant's comfort and privacy. To achieve this, all necessary items should be readily available, including recording equipment, tapes, consent forms, participant information sheets, refreshments, and tissues. Researchers

Table 3.1 Summarizing the key points about effective interviewing techniques

Key aspect	Summary
1. Interview structure	A structured approach is essential for high-quality data; practice sessions or "dummy runs" help refine techniques
2. Preparation	Establish a warm, non-judgmental demeanor, ask balanced questions, choose a suitable setting, and ensure participants are informed about audio/video recording
3. Comfort and privacy	Ensure necessary items are available, minimize disruptions, and arrange the interview room for participant comfort
4. Time management	Allocate enough time for interviews to conclude naturally; focus on gathering participant information without imposing personal views
5. Question techniques	Use structured or semistructured question lists, pay attention to verbal and non-verbal cues, and take detailed notes for analysis
6. Reflection and Memoing	Reflect on the interview process and document unique situations to aid in data analysis
7. Open dialogue	Encourage free expression through techniques like funneling, probing, storytelling, and paraphrasing
8. Language sensitivity	Use respectful and inclusive language, especially in cross-cultural settings, to enhance communication and participant comfort

must proactively minimize potential disruptions by placing "do not disturb" signs and turning off or silencing telephones and pagers. Such measures create an environment conducive to open and uninterrupted communication, facilitating a smoother interview experience for both the participant and the researcher. Additionally, ensuring the interview room is appropriately arranged and that participants are briefed on the process can further enhance their comfort and cooperation.

It is essential to allocate sufficient time for each interview, allowing the conversation to reach its natural conclusion without being rushed or prematurely terminated. The interviewer's active presence and engagement—encompassing attentive listening, thoughtfully attending to responses, and skilfully closing the conversation—are critical to the success of the process. It's important to remember that the interview's primary goal is to elicit information from the participant, not to provide a platform for the researcher's own opinions or feelings.

In structured or semistructured interviews, a well-prepared list of questions is used to guide the conversation. These questions help clarify the discussion for participants who might feel hesitant or confused and can prompt them to provide additional details when needed. Researchers should adopt an active listening stance, paying close attention to both verbal and non-verbal

cues. Some researchers find it beneficial to record non-verbal aspects of the interview through memoing, while others may invite another researcher to take detailed notes during the session. These notes, alongside the audio or video recordings, are invaluable for later analysis.

Moreover, the interviewer should reflect on their thoughts and feelings about the interview and document any unique situations or events that occur. These memos can significantly contribute to a deeper understanding during the data analysis phase, helping to contextualize and interpret the data collected.

Qualitative interviews should be structured to allow interviewees to speak openly, providing in-depth and extended responses. This can be achieved through various techniques, either used individually or combined. Key techniques include:

Funneling: Starting the interview with broad, general questions that are non-threatening, and progressively narrowing the focus to more specific topics as the interview continues [38]. This method helps to ease the participant into the conversation.

Probing: This involves asking for additional details or clarifications to delve deeper into the topic. As detailed by Robinson, [39], the innovative probing technique of "laddered questions" involves a series of questions that progress from the least to the most intrusive. This technique classifies questions from those about "actions" as the least invasive to those about "philosophy"—feelings, values, and beliefs—as the most invasive.

Storytelling: By framing questions in a way that encourages storytelling, interviewees are prompted to provide more elaborate answers [40]. For example, asking "Can you tell me about the last time you experienced…?" invites a narrative response.

Paraphrasing: This technique involves repeating what the participant has said to confirm understanding and clarity, serving as a prompt for further elaboration [36].

It is also crucial to consider the language used during interviews, particularly in cross-cultural contexts. Using language that is respectful, inclusive, and easily understood by participants from diverse backgrounds can significantly enhance communication and ensure that responses are authentic and meaningful. Researchers should be mindful of potential cultural nuances and language barriers, adapting their approach to ensure participants feel comfortable and understood.

3.5.1.3 Advantages of Interviews

Interviews provide researchers with a unique opportunity to gain deep insights into the participant's perspective and to reflect on specific events from their point of view. Building rapport and trust during the interview process is crucial, as it encourages participants to share extensive and detailed information. Ideally, interviews should evolve as conversational exchanges, allowing researchers to clarify topics and explore them in greater depth.

Each interview yields distinct data, as no two participants will provide identical responses. Additionally, interviews offer the flexibility to address sensitive or emotional topics, with the interviewer being equipped to provide appropriate support or refer the participant to counseling services if necessary. Through qualitative interviews, researchers can foster a productive, meaningful, and supportive interaction that benefits both the interviewer and the participant.

Furthermore, interviews enable researchers to capture the nuances of participant responses, including non-verbal cues and emotional undertones, which can be critical for a comprehensive understanding of the subject matter. This method allows for real-time adjustments to the line of questioning, adapting to the flow of the conversation and the participant's comfort level. Such adaptability ensures that the data collected is both rich and relevant.

Interviews also contribute to a collaborative environment where participants feel their perspectives are valued and their contributions are integral to the research. This inclusive approach not only enhances the quality of the data but also empowers participants, providing them with a sense of ownership and investment in the research process. This dynamic often results in more authentic and candid responses, leading to deeper insights and more impactful findings.

3.5.1.4 Disadvantages of Interview

Interviews present various challenges, such as ensuring access to participants, creating sensitive records, and navigating power dynamics, the physical and psychological space, communication nuances, and the sequence of interviews. While the techniques and methods themselves are not the main limitation, their application by researchers often is. Ethically, interview questions must be scrutinized to ensure they are not biased, leading, unbalanced, emotive, imposing, coercive, manipulative, or threatening. It is essential to avoid exacerbating the power imbalance between the interviewer and interviewee. Even with well-planned research designs, some level of power differential in interviews is inevitable. To minimize this, interviewers should explain how answering the questions benefits the participants, thereby helping them feel more in control. A successful interview resembles a conversation rather than a strict question-and-answer session, and interviewers should always treat participants with respect and courtesy.

Interviews can be time-consuming and require significant resources to set up. In qualitative research, estimating the number of interviews needed to collect comprehensive data is an inexact science. Relying solely on single interviews with participants may result in a lack of depth in the information gathered. Additionally, despite efforts to set aside their own experiences, ideas, prejudices, and opinions, interviewers inevitably influence the data to some extent. This influence can manifest through subtle body language, or the way questions are phrased.

Moreover, the logistics of arranging interviews, such as scheduling and finding suitable locations, can pose practical difficulties. The need for interviewer training and the potential for interviewer bias also highlight the importance of preparation and reflexivity. Employing techniques like follow-up interviews or triangulating data sources can help mitigate some of these limitations and enhance the richness and validity of the research findings.

3.5.2   Focus Groups

Focus groups are a valuable method for exploring, developing, and refining initial research questions and interview schedules. Focus groups generally consist of 6–12 members [41]. They play a critical role in forming an evaluative framework that can effectively assess client needs and the outcomes of various investigations. Although focus groups utilize interview schedules, these differ from those in other research interviews due to their unique group dynamics and the rich insights derived from participant interactions. This method provides a collective understanding of the participants' values, experiences, and observations, which are then analyzed within the context of the study. While group synergy or consensus on issues may emerge, it is not always guaranteed [1].

When multiple focus groups are planned, the initial sessions typically aim to identify broad issues and perspectives relevant to the study. Subsequent sessions then focus on prioritizing and narrowing down these identified issues. For example, in a study aimed at enhancing patient care in rural healthcare settings, focus groups were organized with participants who shared common characteristics: they all lived in rural

areas and were regular users of local healthcare services. This approach allowed researchers to address a wide range of concerns affecting patients in these communities, such as accessibility and quality of care.

Furthermore, focus groups can uncover unexpected insights, particularly about the social dynamics and challenges unique to specific demographic groups. The interaction among participants often reveals common challenges and shared solutions that might not surface in one-on-one interviews. The facilitator's role in ensuring balanced discussion is crucial, allowing all participants to contribute and preventing any single individual from dominating the conversation. This balanced approach helps ensure a comprehensive understanding of the issues and contributes to the robustness of the research findings.

3.5.2.1 Advantages of Focus Groups
One of the primary advantages of focus group interviews is that they tend to be less intimidating than one-on-one interviews. This method provides a more comfortable setting for participants who might feel uneasy or apprehensive about individual interviews. The group dynamic fosters supportive interactions, where each member is encouraged to identify, discuss, analyze, and address issues collaboratively.

Focus groups are particularly effective for uncovering new information and gaining diverse perspectives on a topic. They are instrumental in exploring participants' views, beliefs, values, and reasons behind their thoughts and feelings. This approach not only reveals what participants think but also offers insight into why they hold those beliefs.

Additionally, focus group interviews are generally more cost-effective than conducting multiple individual interviews. By gathering a range of opinions in a single session, researchers can obtain a broad spectrum of data while reducing overall expenses and time commitment. This method also allows for the observation of group dynamics, which can provide deeper insights into collective attitudes and experiences. Overall, focus groups offer a valuable opportunity to explore complex topics in a supportive environment, making them a practical and insightful tool for data collection.

3.5.2.2 Disadvantages Focus Groups

Focus groups have certain limitations compared to one-on-one interviews. They may not delve into issues as deeply due to their group format. The less intimate and private nature of focus groups can also make it challenging to uncover sensitive or potentially embarrassing information, as participants might be less inclined to share personal details in a group setting.

Conducting focus group interviews requires a high level of interviewing skill. Researchers need to possess effective "gatekeeping" abilities to manage group dynamics, such as preventing "groupthink" where the consensus may overshadow individual opinions, ensuring no single participant dominates the conversation, and encouraging contributions from quieter members. These skills are essential for maintaining a balanced and productive discussion.

When these challenges are managed effectively, the researcher's role can be minimal, involving primarily starting the discussion, providing occasional prompts, and concluding the session. However, the need for expertise remains crucial to ensure that the focus group yields valuable and balanced insights. Overall, while focus groups offer unique advantages in gathering diverse perspectives, their limitations highlight the importance of skilled facilitation and the potential need for supplementary methods to explore sensitive topics in greater depth.

3.5.3 Observational

Observational methods are frequently utilized in qualitative research designs and exhibit variations depending on the specific method employed. Observation involves closely **watching** participants in their natural environments to document aspects such as social status, roles, actions, and interactions. While qualitative observation is often associated with ethnographers, it is also applicable to a wide array of other qualitative

methodologies (Ref). This method is particularly relevant in studies employing an interpretive or constructivist approach, where analyzing observed events is crucial for interpreting and understanding behaviors (Mulhall).

In qualitative research, observation methods are primarily unstructured, though occasionally some structure may be introduced to align with the research objectives. With unstructured observation, researchers enter the field without a predetermined schedule or specific expectations about what they might encounter. This approach necessitates an "observation protocol" to systematically record information gathered during observations. For example, observers in a hospital ward or clinic may concentrate their observations on a particular phenomenon of interest, ensuring consistent data collection among different observers.

This consistency allows researchers to gain a comprehensive understanding of the context and nuances of the observed behaviors and interactions. By immersing themselves in the natural setting of their subjects, researchers can gather rich, detailed data that might not be accessible through other methods such as interviews or surveys. This method is especially valuable for exploring complex social phenomena and understanding the intricacies of human behavior within specific cultural or social contexts.

Moreover, observation can be a powerful tool for uncovering unspoken norms, hidden patterns, and subtle interactions that might otherwise go unnoticed. It can help researchers identify discrepancies between what people say and what they do, providing a more nuanced and accurate portrayal of their lived experiences. However, this method requires researchers to be mindful of their own biases and the potential influence their presence may have on participants' behavior, thus necessitating careful planning and reflection throughout the research process.

Ultimately, the choice of observational method and the level of structure applied should align with the research questions and objectives, ensuring that the data collected is both meaningful and reliable. As such, observation remains a cornerstone of qualitative research, offering invaluable insights into the complexities of human behavior and social interaction.

3.5.3.1 Conducting the Observation

Observation methods in research span a continuum from participation to observation, with four distinct roles defined within this spectrum: complete participant, participant-as-observer, observer-as-participant, and complete observer. These roles differ primarily in the level of involvement (intervention) or detachment (concealment) the researcher maintains with the participants.

In the role of a complete participant, the researcher is fully integrated as a recognized and established member of the community, group, or sub-group being studied. This immersive involvement affords the researcher an optimal vantage point to observe behaviors as they unfold naturally within the community. This method is commonly employed in anthropological studies, where researchers are either already members of the community or strive to gain acceptance as insiders. Often, community members are unaware that the participant observer is conducting research (a form of concealment), which helps minimize any disruption to the natural activities and dynamics.

In contrast, the participant-as-observer role involves the researcher actively engaging as both participant and observer, but with transparent communication about their dual role. This openness facilitates the development of productive relationships with other participants and grants the researcher the flexibility to enter and exit the research setting as deemed appropriate.

The observer-as-participant role shifts the emphasis to observation, with participation being a secondary concern. Here, the researcher's role as an observer is publicly known, which may limit the establishment of close relationships characteristic of complete participation. However, this role still allows for a nuanced understanding of the research environment through some level of interaction.

Finally, the complete observer role confines the researcher solely to observation without any interaction with the participants. The research study's purpose may or may not be disclosed to those being observed. This approach raises significant ethical concerns, as not informing individuals that they are part of a study can lead to ethical breaches. Consequently, examples of this role are uncommon, not just in nursing and midwifery, but across various disciplines. In some instances, participants may be debriefed after the study's conclusion, but even this delayed disclosure is typically insufficient to secure ethical approval.

Another dimension of observation is the "positioning approach" that the observer adopts, which can be categorized into single, multiple, and mobile positioning. In single positioning, the observer remains in one fixed location throughout the observation period. This strategy minimizes the risk of distracting the participants or the observer being distracted by other elements in the environment, thus allowing for focused data collection.

On the other hand, multiple positioning involves the observer relocating to various spots to capture events from multiple angles or perspectives. This method enables a more comprehensive understanding of the observed phenomena by providing diverse viewpoints. Mobile positioning becomes essential when the observer needs to follow participants as they engage in their daily routines. This approach is particularly useful in dynamic environments where activities are spread out over larger areas, requiring the observer to be adaptable and mobile to capture relevant data.

Video recording is another method of conducting observational studies. The choice of recording method hinges on the research question's focus and the proposed analytical approach. One of the primary advantages of video recording is the ability to replay the footage multiple times, which significantly aids the data analysis process by allowing the researcher to review the events thoroughly. This repeated review can help reduce personal observational bias and ensure a more accurate interpretation of the data.

Moreover, video recording is especially effective in intervention studies, where it can be used to compare pre- and post-intervention practices.

By providing a visual record of changes over time, this method enhances the reliability and validity of the findings, making it a valuable tool for research that seeks to measure the impact of specific interventions.

3.5.3.2 Strength of Observational

There are several benefits to using observation in qualitative research. These include the ability to "capture data in more natural circumstances," allowing researchers to see events and interactions as they naturally unfold without artificial influence (REF). Additionally, observation provides a comprehensive view of the entire social setting and the context in which individuals operate, enabling a deeper understanding of the interactions and dynamics within that environment.

Furthermore, observation sheds light on how the immediate physical environment influences behavior and interactions. By choosing the appropriate observation method, researchers can engage with participants, thereby enriching the data collected with diverse perspectives related to the participants' values and experiences. This interaction not only helps in understanding the participants better but also facilitates the collection of nuanced data that might not be accessible through other research methods.

When the researcher takes on the role of a participant, observation offers a unique opportunity for self-reflection and evaluation of their feelings and experiences within the research setting. This dual role enables researchers to choose whether to "step back from" or "be immersed in" the situations they are observing, allowing for flexibility in their approach to understanding the phenomena under study.

Additionally, this method can contribute to the development of a more empathetic understanding of the participants' experiences, as researchers gain firsthand insights into the challenges and realities faced by those they are studying. The ability to oscillate between observing and participating also helps researchers maintain a balanced perspective, ensuring that their interpretations remain grounded in the observed reality while being informed by their reflective insights. Overall, observation in qualitative research provides a multifaceted approach to data collection, capturing the complexity of human behavior and the subtle influences of environmental factors.

3.5.3.3 Limitation

When conducting research from an "objective" perspective, it is important to acknowledge that observation is often more susceptible to "subjective" interpretation by the researcher compared to interview data. This is partly because field notes, which are frequently documented after the observation event, can contribute to the subjectivity of the data. Nevertheless, these concerns are less significant when working within a constructivist paradigm of research.

Additionally, the Hawthorne effect, or reactivity, is a notable limitation in observational research methods [42]. This phenomenon occurs when individuals aware that they are being studied—particularly through observation—alter their behavior, either to please the researcher or to present themselves in a more favorable light. To mitigate participant "reactivity," one potential solution is to conceal the researcher's role from beginning to end, as suggested by Zahle [43].

However, this approach has its drawbacks. Concealment may lead to a lack of objectivity on the part of the researcher. Moreover, when the researcher's identity is eventually disclosed, it could foster feelings of distrust among group members. The ethical implications of such a strategy are also contentious, as participants are essentially being observed without their informed consent. This ethical dilemma underscores the importance of transparency and trust in the researcher-participant relationship, emphasizing the need for careful consideration of the ethical framework within which observational studies are conducted.

3.5.4   Other Data Collection Techniques

While most qualitative studies rely on interviews or observations for data collection, other methods can also be utilized—either independently or in combination with one another.

3.5.4.1 Journaling

Additionally, participants can keep journals to document their experiences, decision-making processes, or other aspects of the study's focus. Journaling typically occurs shortly after an event or experience, which helps to ensure that the recorded information is accurate and reflective of the participant's immediate reactions.

3.5.4.2 Think-Aloud Technique

Another innovative data collection method is the "think-aloud" technique. In this approach, participants vocalize their reflective thoughts, decision-making processes, or impressions of events and incidents, often using a handheld audio recorder. This technique allows researchers to capture real-time insights into the participants' cognitive processes, which can reveal valuable information about their perceptions and reasoning.

3.5.4.3 Systematic Searching for Indirect Data

A well-established data collection method in qualitative research involves a form of "systematic searching" for relevant stored or displayed items, referred to as indirect data, which can be analyzed later. This search might target historical information, such as archival materials, meeting minutes, biographies, personal and organizational diaries, letters, and personal documents. These sources provide rich, contextual information that can contribute to a deeper understanding of the research topic.

For example, a nursing researcher is investigating the historical development of nursing practices in a particular hospital. They conduct a systematic search of archival materials, such as old hospital records, minutes of nursing board meetings, and personal diaries of retired nurses. These documents provide valuable insights into how nursing roles and responsibilities have evolved over time, shedding light on changes in patient care standards and hospital policies.

3.5.4.4 Artistic Media

The systematic search process can also be applied to various forms of literary and artistic media, including paintings, literature, photography, and video. These forms of indirect data can reveal cultural, social, and individual perspectives that are essential to qualitative research.

For example, in a study exploring the emotional experiences of pediatric oncology nurses, researchers might use photography and video as data collection methods. Nurses are asked to take photographs and record videos that capture their daily work environments or significant moments that illustrate their emotional highs and lows. These visual data are then analyzed by the researchers to understand better the emotional landscape of nursing in high-stress settings. This approach allows for a deeper exploration of how nurses cope with the emotional demands of their profession.

3.5.4.5 Participant-Created Artistic Expressions

In some cases, qualitative researchers go a step further by asking participants to engage in artistic processes, such as creating collages, taking photographs, or performing other creative activities related to the study's focus. This approach not only enriches the data set but also provides participants with an alternative means of expressing their thoughts and experiences.

For example, a nursing study focused on the experiences of patients with chronic pain might invite participants to create collages that represent their pain journeys. By selecting images, words, and colors that symbolize their experiences, patients can communicate the complexities of their pain in a non-verbal format. These collages are then analyzed by the researchers to identify common themes and gain insights into the subjective experience of living with chronic pain.

3.6   Data Analysis

Qualitative analysis is an intensive process that demands a blend of creativity, conceptual awareness, and considerable effort. It is often more intricate and challenging than quantitative analysis, partly due to its less structured nature. While the goal of both qualitative and quantitative data analysis is to organize the data, provide structure, and derive meaningful insights, the approach in qualitative research is distinct. In qualitative studies, data collection and analysis are typically conducted simultaneously, rather than waiting until all data has been gathered. From the very start of data collection, researchers begin the process of identifying significant themes and concepts. This early and ongoing analysis allows for a deeper understanding of the data, guiding subsequent data collection and refining the focus of the research as it progresses.

The analysis of qualitative data is a dynamic and interactive process, particularly when it leans toward the interpretive end of the analytical spectrum. Qualitative researchers usually engage deeply with their data, meticulously examining it and repeatedly reading through it to uncover meaning and achieve a deeper understanding. This iterative process is essential for grasping the nuances of the data.

To support and streamline this complex process, qualitative analysis is bolstered by various tasks that assist in organizing and managing the substantial amount of narrative data. These tasks not only facilitate the analysis but also help ensure that the emerging insights are coherent and well-structured. By systematically arranging and interpreting the data, researchers can more effectively reveal the underlying themes and patterns that contribute to a richer understanding of the research subject.

3.6.1   Transcribing

In qualitative research, the most frequently used textual data come from transcripts of recorded interviews and focus groups. Transcription is a critical element of the qualitative research process, as a verbatim transcript captures participants' exact words, language, and expressions (Table 3.2). This allows researchers to decode behaviors, processes, and the cultural meanings embedded in participants' perspectives. The tran-

Table 3.2 Example for Transcript with Possible Codes

Interviewer (I): Thank you for agreeing to participate in this study. To start, could you tell me about your experience with [**patient-centered care**] in your nursing practice?

Participant (P): Of course. In my role as a nurse, I've always prioritized [**patient-centered care**]. It's not just about [**treating the illness**] but [**understanding the person**] behind the patient. For example, I had a patient last month who was really anxious about a procedure. I took extra time to [**explain everything in detail**], using [**simple language**], and reassured them throughout the process. I think that helped a lot in [**easing their anxiety**]

I: That sounds like a valuable approach. Could you elaborate on how you [**integrate patient-centered care**] into your daily routine?

P: Sure. I make it a point to [**listen to my patients' concerns**] without [**rushing them**]. I also involve them in [**decision-making**] as much as possible, whether it's choosing a treatment option or deciding on their care plan. I believe that when patients feel [**heard and respected**], they are more likely to [**engage in their care**], which ultimately leads to [**better outcomes**]

Possible codes:

1. **Patient-centered care:** This is a central theme and could be a primary code for the entire interview, focusing on practices and attitudes related to this approach
2. **Treating the illness vs. understanding the person:** This could be coded under contrasting themes, such as "biomedical approach" vs. "holistic care"
3. **Explaining in detail:** Could be coded as "communication strategies" or "patient education"
4. **Simple language:** Could fall under "communication strategies" or "patient comprehension"
5. **Easing anxiety:** This might be coded as "emotional support" or "anxiety management"
6. **Listening to concerns:** A possible code could be "active listening" or "patient engagement"
7. **Not rushing them:** Could be coded as "time management" or "quality of care"
8. **Involving in decision-making:** This could be coded as "shared decision-making" or "patient autonomy"
9. **Heard and respected:** This might be a code related to "patient dignity" or "patient satisfaction"
10. **Engage in their care:** This could be coded as "patient involvement" or "patient empowerment"
11. **Better outcomes:** Could be linked to "outcome improvement" or "effectiveness of care"

scription of these recordings often results in a substantial amount of data that requires thorough analysis.

In any study report, it is essential for researchers to detail how the data were recorded during interviews, focus groups, or observations, as well as the methods employed to ensure the accuracy of the transcriptions. Typically, transcripts are created by typing out everything from the recording word for word, including all audible sounds such as laughter, coughing, or pauses.

Advancements in technology have introduced voice-activated computer programs that can generate written records from recordings. However, even when using such software or relying on a professional transcriptionist, researchers must verify the accuracy of the transcripts. This is often done by carefully reading and correcting the transcript while simultaneously listening to the recording. This step is crucial to ensure that the final transcripts are accurate and reflective of the participants' true intent, which is vital for the integrity of the qualitative analysis.

3.6.2   Data Management

Qualitative data analysis typically occurs simultaneously with data collection, necessitating careful planning due to the substantial volume of data generated. When qualitative researchers design a study, they must plan for multiple secure locations to store the data. Often, one of these locations includes an online service or electronic network to manage and safeguard the information. The sheer quantity of data can be overwhelming, as a single 1-h interview might produce several electronic files, such as the transcript, field notes, journals related to coding or analysis, and a demographic form.

Experienced researchers develop a consistent and systematic approach to naming files before data collection even begins. For instance, file names might include the interviewee's name or pseudonym, the date of creation, and the type of document (e.g., transcript or field note). Additional files might also be generated from research team meetings or consultations with experts to address challenges that arise during data collection.

Researchers maintain a detailed record of how each file is named and where it is stored, ensuring easy access during the phases of analysis, interpretation, and dissemination. This meticulous organization is crucial for preventing time wasted searching for files, which can hinder the efficiency and effectiveness of the research process. By planning ahead and keeping their data well-organized, researchers can focus more on deriving meaningful insights from their study.

3.6.3   Coding

Coding involves the process of reading through data, breaking down the text into smaller segments, and assigning a label or code to each segment. These labels serve as a tool for researchers to begin identifying patterns within the data, as they can compare sections of text that share the same codes to explore similarities and differences [44]. A code functions as a symbol or abbreviation used to categorize words or phrases within the data. In traditional methods, codes may be handwritten on a printed transcript. In contrast, within a word processing program or CAQDAS, coding is done by highlighting a section of text and adding a comment in the margin or sidebar.

There are various methods for coding or labeling qualitative data. Some researchers employ a note card system, categorizing key quotes under basic codes. Others may handwrite codes in the margins of their transcripts, organizing them into a complex hierarchy based on a codebook they have developed. Color coding and computer software are additional methods available, but ultimately, researchers develop their own systems to organize the data into manageable units.

Data reduction is a critical component of analysis, requiring researchers to make decisions about which data most accurately represent the overall narrative. As researchers identify patterns or categories that best capture the core elements of the data, these choices become integral to the analysis and interpretation process.

There is no universally correct or perfect method for coding data, and no single approach is inherently wrong. Coding is essentially a personalized filing system, which is why there is no one-size-fits-all technique. Consequently, the expertise and judgment of the qualitative researcher are paramount in qualitative research (Table 3.2).

Traditional **open coding** is a common initial step where researchers group data into categories that appear logical. It is essential for researchers to maintain an audit trail, documenting their evolving thoughts and decisions about the naming and assignment of categories. This record allows them to later review why certain labels were chosen and others were not. Following open coding, **axial coding** further refines the analysis by requiring researchers to compare categories and labels, defining and exploring the relationships among them to develop a more nuanced understanding of the data.

Once the data have been organized through basic coding, [45] recommend that researchers move on to generating categories, themes, and patterns. This next step involves identifying meaningful categories that capture relevant **themes**, recurring ideas, or linguistic patterns, as well as underlying beliefs that connect individuals and contexts. Researchers should explore how different codes might be linked by common themes and identify patterns both across and within these themes.

In this phase, it is crucial for researchers to examine how codes intersect and how themes and patterns relate to one another. The analysis should be conducted with the overarching goal in mind: to accurately reflect the data and provide a comprehensive representation of the story or phenomenon being studied. By doing so, researchers ensure that their findings are grounded in the data and faithfully convey the essence of the research subject.

3.6.4 Computer Software

As computer software has advanced, a growing number of qualitative researchers have begun using computer-assisted qualitative data analysis software (CAQDAS) packages. Software designed for qualitative data analysis is invaluable in managing vast amounts of textual information. The software available today falls into several categories, including word processing, text analysis, grouping and linking, and visualizing relationships. The choice of software depends on the specific needs of the researchers, such as how they plan to display or manage the data.

These tools have transformed the way data analysis and related processes are conducted, allowing researchers to work efficiently at their computers with the ability to print out any section of the project file as needed. CAQDAS has become a widely accepted tool in qualitative research, primarily because it significantly reduces the time required to manage large datasets. This efficiency enables researchers to dedicate more time to the in-depth analysis of their data.

A broad range of CAQDAS packages are available, including popular options such as ATLAS.ti, MAXQDA, and NVIVO. These software programs offer powerful search capabilities that enable researchers to sift through hundreds of pages of text to locate specific data, group information, and create charts and graphs, among many other functions. The extensive features of these tools can significantly streamline the analysis process.

However, researchers must carefully evaluate the features of each program and choose the one that best aligns with their qualitative methods and research objectives. The decision should be based on the specific needs of the study, such as the complexity of data management or the types of analysis required.

In addition to specialized software, qualitative researchers often utilize a variety of tools or apps to manage their data effectively. These supplementary tools can enhance the organization, accessibility, and overall management of the data, ensuring a more efficient and comprehensive analysis process.

Despite these benefits, it is important to recognize that computer software cannot replace the human intuition and reflective thought processes that are crucial for analyzing qualitative data. However, several researchers caution against the risk of allowing these tools to overshadow the critical thinking and conceptual mapping that are essential in qualitative analysis [46, 47]. The researcher must be familiar with the methodologies, research design, and philosophical paradigms of their study to effectively use CAQDAS to their advantage. The reliance on software should complement, not replace, the nuanced understanding that researchers bring to their work.

Although software can be advantageous, qualitative data analysis packages are often challenging to learn and require a significant commitment from researchers to master in order to fully utilize their features. The processes of data entry and coding remain time-consuming and can be quite tedious. However, the most significant benefit of these software tools is their ability to group, compare, and contrast data more efficiently, owing to the improved accessibility once the data have been fully entered. This streamlined access facilitates a more thorough and systematic analysis, enabling researchers to uncover deeper insights.

In addition, these programs are valuable when it comes to preparing written reports, selecting relevant quotations, or condensing data for presentations. Despite this, some researchers prefer to use basic word processing software for these tasks, finding it sufficient depending on the complexity and demands of their project. Ultimately, the choice between advanced software and simpler tools depends on the researcher's specific needs and their proficiency with the technology.

3.6.5 Interpretation

Themes begin to emerge as individual codes are synthesized into more abstract concepts or phrases. Often, these themes develop in layers, with each subsequent layer representing a higher level of abstraction beyond the initial codes. As themes become more abstract, it can become increasingly challenging to maintain clear connections between the themes and the original data. Ensuring the clarity of these links is crucial

for maintaining the rigor of the study. While CAQDAS can automate the creation of these linkages, it is ultimately the researcher's responsibility to ensure that the connections from themes back to codes, and from codes to the original data, are rigorous and accurate.

When critically appraising a qualitative study that utilizes themes, it is important to identify the themes presented, evaluate whether the researcher has provided appropriate participant quotes to support those themes, and assess whether the themes are sufficient and adequately represent the data. During the interpretation phase, the researcher places the findings within a broader context, potentially linking different themes or factors to one another. Interpretation may explore the practical implications of the findings for clinical practice or may delve into theorizing, connecting the study's insights to existing theories or suggesting new theoretical frameworks.

When selecting a narrative style for reporting study results, researchers should prioritize effectively conveying their findings in a manner that resonates with and is easily understood by the intended audience. It is crucial to tailor the report with the readers' needs in mind, ensuring that the presentation of the results is not only informative but also engaging. For example, when the audience consists of nursing students, the report should emphasize foundational concepts and practical applications. In contrast, when addressing registered nurses pursuing their master's degrees, the focus should shift toward advanced theories and critical analysis. Similarly, when the readers are interdisciplinary team members outside of nursing, the report should highlight the broader implications and relevance of the findings across various fields. In all cases, the goal is to craft a report that is both meaningful and accessible, fostering a deeper understanding and application of the research findings.

Reporting formats vary significantly among the four major types of qualitative research, reflecting their distinct objectives and methods. In **phenomenological** research, the goal is to deeply explore and convey the lived experiences of participants. This approach often benefits from a narrative style that is rich and descriptive, capturing the essence of these experiences in a way that resonates with readers. While a realist voice can effectively present detailed descriptions and interpretations, an evocative, impressionistic style might offer a more immersive and emotionally engaging portrayal.

Grounded theory is typically reported in a more traditional and analytical manner, focusing on presenting the processes and theories developed by the researcher. This approach usually requires a detached, analytic style of reporting. Regardless of the narrative style chosen, it is crucial to tailor the report to the specific audience and select the most effective method for communication.

In **ethnographic** research, researchers often use a realist voice, but an impressionistic approach might be more suitable for conveying concepts related to different cultures. For instance, when studying the death and burial practices of a remote tribe, a storytelling approach may offer a richer and more engaging presentation of the findings.

In **historical** research, the realist voice is commonly employed because the data are usually derived from historical documents. These documents can serve both as commentary and evidence in qualitative research. When using documents as primary data sources, reports might include more detailed discussion and observation. Nevertheless, researchers may choose a different voice or a more creative reporting approach to enhance the presentation of the results.

3.6.6 Artificial Intelligence

Artificial Intelligence (AI) has increasingly become a transformative tool across various fields, including the analysis of qualitative data in research. Qualitative research, which focuses on understanding human experiences, behaviors, and social phenomena, traditionally involves the manual analysis of non-numerical data such as interviews, focus group discussions, and open-ended survey responses. The advent of AI has introduced new possibilities for enhancing the

efficiency, consistency, and depth of qualitative data analysis.

Two leading software packages for qualitative data analysis, ATLAS.ti [48] and MAXQDA [49], have both formed partnerships with OpenAI, the organization behind ChatGPT. ATLAS.ti has integrated AI into its platform with a focus on automatic coding, which leverages AI to identify and categorize themes in the data without the need for user-initiated queries. This approach contrasts with more traditional methods, were researchers manually code data or query specific segments for analysis. The incorporation of AI in these software packages reflects a broader trend in qualitative research toward automating complex processes, thereby enabling researchers to handle larger datasets with greater efficiency and consistency. MAXQDA, while also benefiting from AI capabilities, may offer different features or approaches to AI integration, highlighting the diverse ways in which these tools can enhance qualitative research practices.

One of the primary applications of AI in qualitative research is in the automation of data coding. Traditionally, researchers manually code qualitative data by identifying and categorizing themes, patterns, and concepts. AI, through natural language processing (NLP) algorithms, can assist in this process by automatically identifying themes and patterns in large datasets. Machine learning models can be trained to recognize specific topics or sentiments within the data, enabling researchers to code data more quickly and consistently. This automation not only saves time but also reduces the potential for human error and bias in the coding process.

Beyond coding, AI can assist in the interpretation of qualitative data. Advanced AI systems can perform sophisticated text analysis, such as sentiment analysis, topic modeling, and even discourse analysis. These techniques allow researchers to uncover deeper insights from the data, such as underlying emotions, attitudes, or social dynamics that may not be immediately apparent through manual analysis. AI can also help in comparing large volumes of text across different datasets, revealing patterns and trends that would be difficult to detect manually.

Despite its potential, AI in qualitative research is not without limitations. AI systems are only as good as the data and algorithms that underpin them. The nuanced and context-dependent nature of qualitative data means that AI may not always capture the full richness of human experiences [50, 51]. Therefore, AI should be viewed as a tool that complements, rather than replaces, the expertise and judgment of human researchers.

3.7   Trustworthiness

All research aims to produce valid and reliable knowledge ethically, which is crucial for ensuring the trustworthiness of findings, especially in nursing, where practitioners directly intervene in people's lives. Trustworthiness in qualitative research refers to the quality, authenticity, and truthfulness of the findings. It reflects the extent to which readers can trust or have confidence in the results.

In their seminal work during the 1980s, Guba and Lincoln replaced the traditional concepts of reliability and validity in qualitative research with the parallel concept of "trustworthiness" [52–54]. This concept comprises four key aspects: credibility, transferability, dependability, and confirmability. Later, in response to critiques and the evolution of their thinking, [55] added a fifth criterion, authenticity, which is more closely aligned with the constructivist paradigm. To ensure qualitative rigor, Guba and Lincoln introduced methodological strategies such as creating an audit trail, conducting member checks, engaging in peer debriefing, performing negative case analysis, ensuring structural corroboration, and using referential material adequacy [56].

3.7.1   Credibility

In qualitative research, credibility is comparable to internal validity in quantitative research. It denotes the degree of confidence in the accuracy and trustworthiness of the data and its interpretations. To establish and assess credibility, researchers should employ well-established methods and

provide detailed descriptions of their procedures to allow for replication. If similar studies using different methods yield consistent results, it reinforces the credibility of the original findings. Additionally, incorporating feedback from participants and peers can further enhance credibility, ensuring that the research findings are robust and reflective of the studied phenomenon.

3.7.1.1 Prolonged Engagement
A crucial first step in qualitative research is prolonged engagement, which involves dedicating adequate time to collecting data in order to gain a thorough understanding of the culture, language, or perspectives of the group being studied. This approach helps identify and correct misinformation and distortions while also fostering trust and rapport with informants. Building such relationships is essential for obtaining valuable, accurate, and comprehensive information.

3.7.1.2 Persistent Observation
Credible data collection in naturalistic inquiries requires persistent observation. This process involves maintaining a focus on the significant aspects of the data being gathered and recorded. Persistent observation ensures that researchers concentrate on the elements of a situation or conversation that are most relevant to the phenomena being investigated. By doing so, researchers can capture the nuances and details essential for a deep and accurate understanding of the research topic.

3.7.1.3 Debriefing
Debriefing is a critical process in qualitative research that involves presenting and discussing research findings with colleagues or peers. This practice serves several important purposes: it helps prevent researcher bias, aids in the conceptual development of the study, and enhances the overall rigor of the research. This practice is particularly beneficial for novice investigators. Peer debriefing, specifically, offers researchers the opportunity to gain insights and feedback from a professional colleague. The peer providing feedback should have similar educational qualifications and professional standing as the researcher

but should not hold a supervisory or authoritative role. This ensures that the feedback is constructive and unbiased, promoting a more thorough and objective evaluation of the research data.

3.7.1.4 Member Check

Another key strategy for ensuring credibility in qualitative research is member checks, also known as **respondent validation** [2]. This approach involves seeking feedback on your emerging findings from some of the participants. Member checks are one of the most effective methods for eliminating the possibility of misinterpreting the participants' words, actions, and perspectives. This strategy also helps identify any biases or misunderstandings you may have developed during your observations.

The process of conducting member checks involves taking your preliminary analysis back to a selection of participants and asking them whether your interpretation resonates with their experience. Although your interpretation may use different wording—since it is your analysis based on their experiences—participants should still recognize their experiences in your interpretation. They may also suggest adjustments to better align the interpretation with their perspectives.

3.7.1.5 Negative Case Analysis

Negative case analysis is crucial for understanding the norm, or the most commonly occurring cases, in qualitative research [15]. Unlike in quantitative research, where outliers might be disregarded, negative cases are not ignored. Instead, they are examined just as thoroughly as the more frequent cases. Additional cases are also sought out and compared to ensure that the data, including negative cases, is fully saturated.

What does it mean to say that negative cases are "the key to understanding the norm"? [57]. By comparing negative cases with more typical cases, researchers can uncover significant differences. Understanding these differences is often essential for gaining a comprehensive understanding of the overall process. This makes negative case analysis a vital strategy for enhancing the validity of qualitative research.

3.7.1.6 Triangulation

Triangulation is another method that can enhance credibility in qualitative research. As previously mentioned, triangulation involves using multiple sources or methods to draw conclusions about what constitutes truth, and it has been likened to convergent validation [2]. The purpose of triangulation is to mitigate the inherent biases that can arise from relying on a single method, observer, or theory. Additionally, triangulation has been argued to provide a more comprehensive and contextualized understanding of the phenomenon under study—an objective shared by researchers across all qualitative traditions. Denzin [58] identified four types of triangulations: data triangulation, investigator triangulation, method triangulation, and theory triangulation.

3.7.1.7 Data Triangulation

Data triangulation involves using multiple data sources to validate research conclusions. There are three primary types of data triangulation: time, space, and person [59]. **Time triangulation** entails collecting data on the same phenomenon or from the same individuals at different points in time. This can include gathering data at various times of the day or during different seasons. The goal is not to study the phenomenon longitudinally to observe changes but to assess the consistency of the phenomenon across different times, similar to a test-retest reliability assessment. **Space triangulation** involves gathering data on the same phenomenon across multiple locations, aiming to validate the findings by checking for consistency across different sites. Finally, **person triangulation** refers to collecting data from different levels of people, such as individuals, groups (like dyads, triads, or families), and larger collectives (such as organizations, communities, or institutions). The purpose here is to validate the data by examining the phenomenon from multiple perspectives.

Investigator Triangulation

Investigator triangulation involves having two or more researchers analyze and interpret the same data set [60]. Collaborating in this way helps minimize the risk of biased data interpretation.

Additionally, when investigators bring a complementary mix of skills and expertise to the analysis, the interpretation benefits from diverse perspectives. The integration of different methodological, disciplinary, and clinical skills can also enhance other forms of triangulation. Conceptually, investigator triangulation is somewhat analogous to interrater reliability in quantitative research.

Theory Triangulation
Theory triangulation involves researchers using different theories or hypotheses to analyze and interpret their data [2]. Qualitative researchers who develop alternative hypotheses while still in the field can test the validity of each, thanks to the flexible design of qualitative studies, which allows for continuous adjustments to the inquiry. This approach helps researchers rule out competing hypotheses and avoid premature conclusions. The quantitative equivalent of theory triangulation is construct validation.

Method Triangulation
Method triangulation involves employing multiple data collection methods to explore the same phenomenon [2]. In qualitative research, this often includes a diverse mix of unstructured methods, such as interviews, observations, and document analysis, to gain a comprehensive understanding of the phenomenon. Utilizing multiple methods allows researchers to assess whether a consistent and cohesive picture of the phenomenon emerges.

3.7.1.8 Reflexivity
The integrity of the qualitative researcher is often referred to as researcher's position or, more recently, reflexivity. This strategy involves critically reflecting on oneself as a researcher—the "human as instrument" [61]. Investigators should articulate their biases, dispositions, and assumptions about the research to be conducted. Even in journal articles, authors are increasingly expected to clarify their assumptions, experiences, worldview, and theoretical orientation regarding the study. This clarification helps readers understand how the researcher's perspectives might have influenced their interpretation of the data. As [62]

notes, the goal of making one's perspective, biases, and assumptions explicit is not to eliminate differences in values and expectations among researchers, but to understand how these values and expectations shape the conduct and conclusions of the study.

3.7.2 Transferability

Transferability refers to the extent to which research findings can be generalized to other settings or groups. This aspect is primarily tied to the study's sampling and design rather than the intrinsic quality of the data. Nonetheless, as [54] emphasize, it is the investigator's duty to provide detailed descriptions in the research report, allowing others to evaluate the relevance of the findings to different contexts. They argue that a researcher cannot directly establish the external validity of a study; instead, they can offer a thorough description that enables others to decide if the findings can be transferred. Such thick description includes a comprehensive and detailed account of the research environment, as well as the interactions and processes observed during the study. Therefore, for transferability to be considered, the researcher must provide enough information to support informed judgments about the comparability of different contexts.

3.7.3 Dependability

In qualitative research, dependability is comparable to reliability in quantitative research. It indicates that the study's findings should remain consistent over time, with a sufficient number of observations to demonstrate this consistency. Dependability is reinforced when coding checks reveal agreement both within and across the identified concepts and themes. Additionally, linking new findings to existing theories can further enhance dependability. Peer review or debriefing by colleagues also supports the study's dependability. There should be a logical coherence between participants' responses, which should be reflected in the coding and analysis processes. An audit trail is essential to demonstrate the rigor of the research method, with multiple journals used to document thoughts, decisions, and reflections on the data and coding procedures.

3.7.4 Confirmability

Confirmability in qualitative research is akin to objectivity in quantitative research. It emphasizes the neutrality of the research findings rather than the researcher [4]. While some subjectivity is inherent in qualitative methods, as the researcher serves as the primary instrument for data collection, analysis, and interpretation, confirmability is questioned when potential biases are not recognized or accounted for. To ensure researchers stay true to the data, techniques such as member checks and peer debriefing can be employed. A thorough description of the study's methods, accompanied by a detailed audit trail, is essential. Researchers should also maintain reflective journals, accurately record all data, and ensure the findings appear genuine and credible.

3.7.5 Authenticity

Authenticity in research reflects the degree to which researchers accurately and impartially present a diverse range of realities [55]. It is evident in a report that captures the emotional tone of participants' lives as they are truly lived. A text is considered authentic if it immerses readers in a vicarious experience of these lives, allowing them to gain a deeper sensitivity to the issues being explored. When authenticity is achieved, readers can better understand the lives portrayed, appreciating the mood, experiences, language, and context in a holistic way [63].

References

1. Patton MQ. Qualitative research & evaluation methods: integrating theory and practice. Thousand Oaks: SAGE; 2023.
2. Denzin NK, Lincoln YS, Giardina MD, Cannella GS. The SAGE handbook of qualitative research. Thousand Oaks: SAGE; 2023.
3. Tesch R. Qualitative research: analysis types and software. New York: Routledge; 2016.
4. Creswell JW, Poth CN. Qualitative inquiry and research design: choosing among five approaches. Thousand Oaks: SAGE; 2024.
5. Husserl E. Ideas: general introduction to pure phenomenology. London: Taylor & Francis; 2015.
6. van Manen M, van Manen M. Doing phenomenological research and writing. Qual Health Res. 2021;31:1069–82. https://doi.org/10.1177/10497323211003058.
7. Collins CS, Stockton CM. The central role of theory in qualitative research. Int J Qual Methods. 2018;17 https://doi.org/10.1177/1609406918797475.
8. van Manen M. Phenomenology of practice: meaning-giving methods in phenomenological research and writing. London: Taylor & Francis; 2023.
9. Heidegger M. Introduction to phenomenological research. Bloomington: Indiana University Press; 2005.
10. Al-Sheikh Hassan M. The use of Husserl's phenomenology in nursing research: a discussion paper. J Adv Nurs. 2023;79:3160–9. https://doi.org/10.1111/jan.15564.
11. Glaser BG, Strauss AL. The discovery of grounded theory: strategies for qualitative research. Chicago: Aldine; 1967.
12. Connor J, Flenady T, Massey D, Dwyer T. Classic grounded theory: identifying the main concern. Res Nurs Health. 2024;47:277–88. https://doi.org/10.1002/nur.22381.
13. Didier A, Nathaniel A, Scott H, et al. Protecting personhood: a classic grounded theory. Qual Health Res. 2023;33:1177–88. https://doi.org/10.1177/10497323231190329.
14. Holloway I, Galvin K. Qualitative research in nursing and healthcare. New York: Wiley; 2023.
15. Flick U. An introduction to qualitative research. Thousand Oaks: SAGE; 2023.
16. Wehbe-Alamah H, McFarland M. Leininger's ethnonursing research method: historical retrospective and overview. J Transcult Nurs. 2020;31:337–49. https://doi.org/10.1177/1043659620912308.
17. Tappen RM. Advanced nursing research: from theory to practice: from theory to practice. 3rd ed. Burlington: Jones & Bartlett Learning; 2022.
18. Crabtree BF, Miller WL. Doing qualitative research. Thousand Oaks: SAGE; 2023.
19. Cabote C, Salamonson Y, Ramjan L, et al. The synergy of critical realism and case study: a novel approach in nursing research. Int J Qual Methods. 2024;23 https://doi.org/10.1177/16094069241254010.
20. deMarrais K, Roulston K, Copple J. Qualitative research design and methods: an introduction. Gorham: Myers Education Press; 2023.
21. Garvey CM, Jones R. Is there a place for theoretical frameworks in qualitative research? Int J Qual Methods. 2021;20 https://doi.org/10.1177/1609406920987959.

22. Savin-Baden M, Major CH. Qualitative research: the essential guide to theory and practice. London: Taylor & Francis; 2023.
23. CohenMiller A. Transformative moments in qualitative research: method, theory, and reflection. London: Taylor & Francis; 2023.
24. Nguyen TNM, Whitehead L, Dermody G, Saunders R. The use of theory in qualitative research: challenges, development of a framework and exemplar. J Adv Nurs. 2022;78:e21–8. https://doi.org/10.1111/jan.15053.
25. Rahimi S, Khatooni M. Saturation in qualitative research: an evolutionary concept analysis. Int J Nurs Stud Adv. 2024;6:100174. https://doi.org/10.1016/j.ijnsa.2024.100174.
26. Hennink MM, Kaiser BN, Marconi VC. Code saturation versus meaning saturation: how many interviews are enough? Qual Health Res. 2017;27:591–608. https://doi.org/10.1177/1049732316665344.
27. Hennink M, Kaiser BN. Sample sizes for saturation in qualitative research: a systematic review of empirical tests. Soc Sci Med. 2022;292:114523. https://doi.org/10.1016/j.socscimed.2021.114523.
28. Naeem M, Ozuem W, Howell K, Ranfagni S. Demystification and actualisation of data saturation in qualitative research through thematic analysis. Int J Qual Methods. 2024;23:1–17. https://doi.org/10.1177/16094069241229777.
29. Tight M. Saturation: an overworked and misunderstood concept? Qual Inq. 2023;30:577. https://doi.org/10.1177/10778004231183948.
30. DiStefano AS, Yang JS. Sample size and saturation: a three-phase method for ethnographic research with multiple qualitative data sources. Field Methods. 2024;36:145–59. https://doi.org/10.1177/1525822X231194515.
31. Guest G, Namey E, Chen M. A simple method to assess and report thematic saturation in qualitative research. PLoS One. 2020;15:e0232076. https://doi.org/10.1371/journal.pone.0232076.
32. Bartholomew TT, Joy EE, Kang E, Brown J. A choir or cacophony? Sample sizes and quality of conveying participants' voices in phenomenological research. Methodol Innov. 2021;14 https://doi.org/10.1177/20597991211040063.
33. Dodgson JE. Phenomenology: researching the lived experience. J Hum Lact. 2023;39:385–96. https://doi.org/10.1177/08903344231176453.
34. Conlon C, Timonen V, Elliott-O'Dare C, et al. Confused about theoretical sampling? Engaging theoretical sampling in diverse grounded theory studies. Qual Health Res. 2020;30:947–59. https://doi.org/10.1177/1049732319899139.
35. Olmo-Extremera M, Fernández-Terol L, Amber Montes D. Visual tools for supporting interviews in qualitative research: new approaches. Qual Res J. 2023;24:283–98. https://doi.org/10.1108/QRJ-07-2023-0113.
36. Edwards R, Holland J. Qualitative interviewing: research methods. London: Bloomsbury Publishing; 2023.
37. Demirci JR. About research: conducting better qualitative interviews. J Hum Lact. 2024;40:21–4. https://doi.org/10.1177/08903344231213651.
38. Pitney W, Parker J, Mazerolle S, Potteiger K. Qualitative research in the health professions. London: Taylor & Francis; 2024.
39. Robinson OC. Probing in qualitative research interviews: theory and practice. Qual Res Psychol. 2023;20:382–97. https://doi.org/10.1080/14780887.2023.2238625.
40. Privitera GJ. Research methods for the behavioral sciences. Thousand Oaks: SAGE; 2024.
41. Geampana A, Perrotta M. Using interview excerpts to facilitate focus group discussion. Qual Res. 2024; https://doi.org/10.1177/14687941241234283.
42. Jianmin S. Hawthorne Experiment. The ECPH Encyclopedia of Psychology [Internet]. Springer, Singapore; 2024 [cited 2024 Dec 2]. p. 1–1. Available from: https://link.springer.com/referenceworkentry/10.1007/978-981-99-6000-2_768-1.
43. Zahle J. Reactivity and good data in qualitative data collection. Euro Jnl Phil Sci. 2023;13(1):10.
44. Stevens PAJ. Qualitative data analysis: key approaches. Thousand Oaks: SAGE; 2022.
45. Marshall C, Rossman GB, Blanco GL. Designing qualitative research. Thousand Oaks: SAGE; 2022.
46. Gupta A. Codes and Coding. In: Gupta A, editor. Qualitative Methods and Data Analysis Using ATLAS.ti: A Comprehensive Researchers' Manual [Internet]. Cham: Springer International Publishing; 2023 [cited 2024 Aug 17]. p. 99–125. Available from: https://doi.org/10.1007/978-3-031-49650-9_4.
47. Reyes V, Bogumil E, Welch LE. The living codebook: documenting the process of qualitative data analysis. Sociological Methods & Research. SAGE Publications Inc. 2024;1;53(1):89–120.
48. ATLAS.ti. AI coding powered by OpenAI. ATLAS.ti; 2024. https://atlasti.com/ai-coding-powered-by-openai. Accessed 18 Aug 2024.
49. MAXQDA. Utilizing the power of AI in qualitative data analysis. MAXQDA; 2024. https://www.maxqda.com/products/ai-assist. Accessed 18 Aug 2024.
50. Hitch D. Artificial intelligence augmented qualitative analysis: the way of the future? Qual Health Res. 2024;34:595–606. https://doi.org/10.1177/10497323231217392.
51. Morgan DL. Exploring the use of artificial intelligence for qualitative data analysis: the case of ChatGPT. Int J Qual Methods. 2023;22:1–10. https://doi.org/10.1177/16094069231211248.
52. Guba EG, Lincoln YS. Epistemological and methodological bases of naturalistic inquiry.

ECTJ. 1982;30:233–52. https://doi.org/10.1007/BF02765185.

53. Guba EG, Lincoln YS. Effective evaluation: improving the usefulness of evaluation results through responsive and naturalistic approaches. San Francisco: Jossey-Bass; 1981.

54. Lincoln YS, Guba EG. Naturalistic inquiry. SAGE; 1985.

55. Guba EG, Lincoln YS. Competing paradigms in qualitative research. In: Handbook of qualitative research. Thousand Oaks: SAGE; 1994. p. 105–17.

56. Lincoln YS, Guba EG. But is it rigorous? Trustworthiness and authenticity in naturalistic evaluation. New Dir Program Eval. 1986;1986:73–84. https://doi.org/10.1002/ev.1427.

57. Morse JM. Critical analysis of strategies for determining rigor in qualitative inquiry. Qual Health Res. 2015;25:1212–22. https://doi.org/10.1177/1049732315588501.

58. Denzin NK. The research act: a theoretical introduction to sociological methods. Hoboken: Prentice Hall; 1989.

59. Denzin NK. The research act: a theoretical introduction to sociological methods. New York: Routledge; 2017.

60. Tisdell EJ, Merriam SB. Qualitative research: a guide to design and implementation. New York: Wiley; 2025.

61. Jamieson MK, Govaart GH, Pownall M. Reflexivity in quantitative research: a rationale and beginner's guide. Soc Personal Psychol Compass. 2023;17:e12735. https://doi.org/10.1111/spc3.12735.

62. Maxwell JA. Qualitative research design. Thousand Oaks: SAGE; 2020.

63. Polit D, Beck C. Essentials of nursing research: appraising evidence for nursing practice. 10th ed. Philadelphia: LWW; 2021.

Mixed Methods in Nursing Research

4

Learning Outcomes

By the end of this chapter, you will be able to:

1. Understand the fundamental principles and components of mixed-methods research in nursing.
2. Explain the philosophical foundations of mixed-methods research, including pragmatism and its role in guiding research design.
3. Differentiate between convergent, explanatory sequential, exploratory sequential, and embedded mixed-methods designs.
4. Analyze the factors that influence the integration of quantitative and qualitative data in mixed-methods research.
5. Evaluate the challenges and strategies for ensuring the validity and reliability of mixed-methods research findings.

4.1 Introduction

Nursing research is often defined by its inherent complexity, which is evident in the multifaceted nature of nursing systems, the challenges they present, and the solutions they require. This complexity is characterized by a continuously evolving set of processes and elements that not only interact but are also mutually shaped by these interactions. As our comprehension of nursing systems and their challenges has progressed, the demand for novel methods and tools to address new research questions has intensified. As a result, researchers are compelled to continuously refine their strategies to effectively engage with the ever-changing field of nursing research. In response to these challenges, many researchers have embraced a mixed-methods approach, integrating both quantitative and qualitative techniques within a single study. Originating in the late 1970s, mixed-methods research leverages numerical data alongside qualitative insights, offering a richer, more nuanced understanding of various aspects of a research question, particularly in the context of nursing [1]. This approach enables researchers to draw more robust and well-rounded conclusions, ultimately enhancing the quality of nursing research.

Mixed-methods research is a developing methodology that systematically combines quantitative and qualitative approaches to address research questions comprehensively. Creswell and Creswell [2] defines mixed-methods research as involving at least one quantitative strand and one qualitative strand. A strand represents a segment of the study characterized by the research process, which includes posing a research question, selecting methods, and collecting and analyzing data. The integration of quantitative and qualitative data throughout the research process is essential to mixed-methods research [3]. This approach allows researchers to leverage the strengths of both numerical data and narrative insights to address different facets or stages of a research question.

Blending data from different sources, mixed-methods research provides a more holistic understanding of the research problem, helping to mitigate the limitations inherent in using a single method. This approach offers both a deep and broad perspective on the issues being studied, enriching the overall findings. As a result, mixed-methods research has become increasingly valuable in nursing, where understanding complex, multifaceted problems requires both quantitative precision and qualitative depth.

4.2   Philosophical Grounding of Mixed-Methods Research

Research studies are typically guided by one or more paradigms, which represent the researchers' fundamental philosophical perspectives on truth, reality, and the specific issues under investigation. These paradigms reflect the philosophical stance researchers take on the nature of reality and the methods used to understand it, encompassing assumptions about ontology (the nature of being) and epistemology (the nature of knowledge), which shape the overall research approach (Fig. 4.1).

Depending on their research goals, researchers may adopt various methods to uncover truths or generate knowledge. Mixed-methods research is a methodology that combines multiple approaches to address research questions in a comprehensive and systematic way. It involves the collection, analysis, interpretation, and reporting of both qualitative and quantitative data. By integrating different methods, mixed-methods research offers a more holistic perspective and deeper insights into complex research questions, allowing for a more nuanced understanding of the phenomena under study.

Mixed-methods research emerged as a distinct approach within the social and behavioral sciences, arising from the earlier dominance of

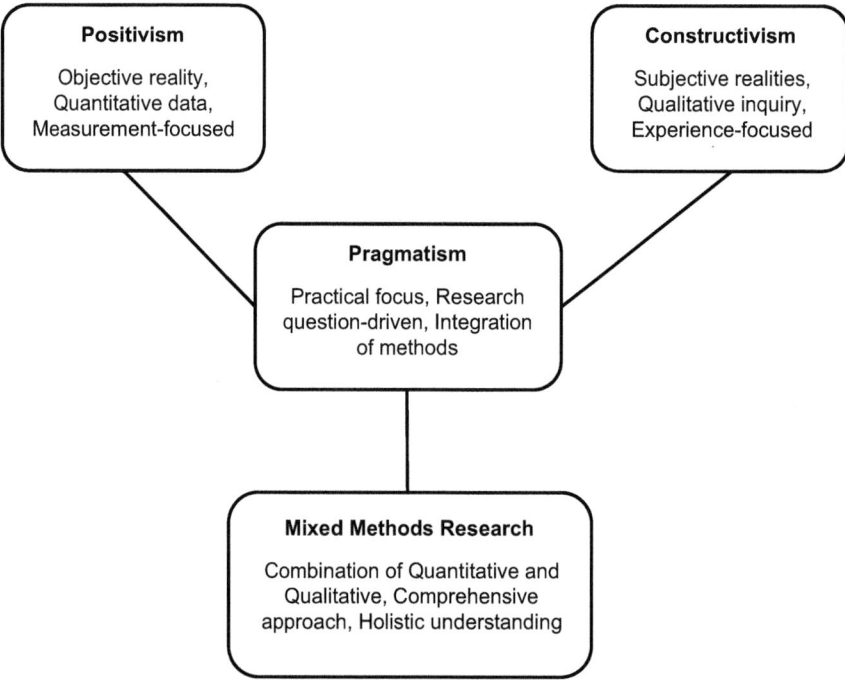

Fig. 4.1 Evolution of research paradigms leading to mixed-methods design

quantitative and qualitative methodologies, each rooted in different paradigms: positivism and constructivism, respectively. The positivist paradigm posits a single, objective reality that can be measured and understood through quantitative data. In contrast, the constructivist paradigm emphasizes the construction of reality through human experiences, acknowledging multiple, subjective realities that are explored through qualitative inquiry.

For a time, these paradigms were often in conflict, leading to the 'paradigm wars,' which positioned them as opposing ways of understanding and studying reality. However, methodological scholars began to recognize that integrating both quantitative and qualitative approaches within a single study could significantly enhance research outcomes, leading to a shift toward a more integrative approach.

From these debates, a third philosophical perspective, pragmatism, emerged. Pragmatism provides a framework that allows researchers to integrate both quantitative and qualitative methods to address research questions effectively. Pragmatists argue that the research question should guide the entire process, advocating for the use of the most suitable methods for the specific problem at hand. They believe that while an objective reality exists, it can only be fully understood through interaction with the environment.

Mixed-methods research is deeply rooted in this pragmatic philosophy, emphasizing the importance of focusing on research questions and outcomes rather than being confined to specific methods. This approach is particularly advantageous in health policy and systems research, where it is crucial to explore "why" and "how" questions alongside "what" questions. For instance, a nurse researcher might investigate whether a new patient education program improves adherence to medication regimens among patients with chronic conditions, and if so, explore how and why it enhances adherence. Addressing these "how" and "why" questions is essential in health systems and implementation research, as it provides insights that can be broadly applied.

4.3 Essential Factors in Mixed Methods

A research design is a deliberate structure that defines the strategy and methods used to address the research question. The formulation of research questions plays a critical role in shaping the specific research design chosen. Research questions that require a mixed-methods approach inherently involve diverse elements, needing quantitative data for some aspects and qualitative insights for others. These questions can be framed either as a single overarching question that demands both types of data or as multiple questions, each requiring different approaches. As a result, various mixed-methods designs may emerge, and the number of potential purposes for mixing methods is vast and continues to grow, making it impossible to provide a comprehensive list of all possibilities.

From a nursing perspective, crafting a mixed-methods design requires careful consideration of several key factors to ensure the study is cohesive and effective. These factors shape the overall research process and influence how data is collected, analyzed, and interpreted. The four essential elements of mixed-method design that will be discussed are: **Theoretical Perspective, Priority of Research Strategy, Sequence of Data Collection**, and **Integration of Data**. These elements are vital in shaping the development of a well-structured mixed-methods approach, especially in the context of nursing research.

4.3.1 Theoretical Perspective

A theoretical perspective plays an integral role in mixed-methods studies, guiding the selection of a specific research design and shaping the overall research process. This perspective can draw from a wide range of theories, from formal empirical theories to epistemological frameworks, social theories, or theoretical propositions related to socioeconomic, cultural, or lifestyle factors. The theoretical perspective can be explicit, meaning it is firmly based on a specific, well-defined theory, or implicit, where the research is indirectly influenced by broader theoretical ideas. Mixed-methods design driven by a theoretical framework are often referred to as transformative designs, as the theory helps to frame not only the methodology but also the interpretation of the findings. Incorporating a theoretical perspective ensures that the research approach is aligned with broader conceptual frameworks, whether explicitly or implicitly, thereby enhancing the depth and relevance of the study.

4.3.2 Priority of Research Strategy

The priority given to quantitative or qualitative components is largely determined by how the research question is framed. Priority refers to the relative emphasis placed on either the qualitative or quantitative aspects of the study. In some cases, equal weight may be given to both qualitative and quantitative components, allowing for a balanced exploration of the research question from both perspectives. In exploratory research, where concepts, variables, and relationships are unclear, greater priority is often assigned to qualitative methods, with quantitative analysis used later to further investigate these relationships. On the other hand, in explanatory research, where findings from a population-level survey are the focus, the quantitative component typically takes precedence, with qualitative methods used to support or contextualize the results.

The combination of sequence and priority in both qualitative and quantitative data collection and analysis results in different types of mixed-methods studies, offering flexibility to adapt the research design to the specific nature of the study. This flexibility ensures that the approach aligns with the research questions and objectives, providing a comprehensive understanding of the topic Table 4.1.

4.3.3 Sequence of Data Collection

In designing mixed-methods research, the sequence of qualitative and quantitative data collection is a crucial consideration, closely aligned with the research question. The way the research question is framed determines whether the quantitative strand should occur before, after, or concurrently with the qualitative strand. There are three main sequence options: qualitative first, quantitative first, or no sequence where both occur simultaneously.

In qualitative first designs, also known as **exploratory sequential** designs, the qualitative strand is conducted first to uncover insights that are then tested or further explored through quantitative methods. In quantitative first designs, also referred to as **explanatory sequential** designs, the quantitative strand is carried out initially, with the qualitative component following to provide deeper explanations for the quantitative findings.

In the case of no sequence, or concurrent designs, both qualitative and quantitative strands are conducted simultaneously, in **parallel**, allowing for the integration of data at various stages of the research. These sequence options provide flexibility, enabling researchers to align the data collection process with the nature of the research question, ensuring that each strand informs and complements the other, ultimately enriching the overall findings.

Table 4.1 Priority in mixed-methods research

Priority	Research type	Focus
Equal	Balanced focus on both	Both qualitative and quantitative components are given equal weight
Qualitative	Exploratory research	Greater emphasis on qualitative methods, with quantitative analysis following
Quantitative	Explanatory research	Quantitative analysis takes precedence, supported by qualitative insights

4.3.4 Integration of Data

Every true mixed-methods study includes at least one "point of integration," also known as the "point of interface," where the qualitative and quantitative components are brought together [4]. This integration point is a defining characteristic of mixed-methods research, distinguishing it from designs that merely use multiple methods. It is at this integration point that the different components are combined, giving rise to the term "mixed-methods design." However, the term "mixing" can be misleading, as it implies a simple blending, when in fact the components must be carefully integrated to ensure coherence and alignment.

True mixed-methods research involves intentional integration at various stages of the research process, whether during **data collection, data analysis, data interpretation**, or through a **combination of these stages**. Integration typically occurs in one of three ways: (1) **merging or converging** the two datasets, often by quantifying qualitative findings; (2) **connecting** the datasets so that the findings of one method inform or are further explored by the other; or (3) **embedding** one dataset within the other, where one type of data plays a supportive role to the primary dataset.

It is not sufficient to simply collect and analyze qualitative and quantitative data separately; they must be intentionally mixed at one or more of these stages to create a more comprehensive understanding than either method could provide alone. The decision regarding when and how to integrate the data—whether at data collection, analysis, interpretation, or through a combination—should be directly tied to the research question and objectives. Integration should not be an afterthought but an integral part of the study design, serving as a pivotal step that enhances the depth and breadth of the research. A well-planned integration process ensures that the strengths of both qualitative and quantitative methods are leveraged effectively, resulting in richer, more nuanced findings.

4.4 Mixed-Methods Design

Mixed-methods designs have evolved into a wide array of types and frameworks, which can often be overwhelming for both novice and experienced mixed-methods researchers. Some of these designs are highly intricate, leading to a growing call for researchers to simplify their approach by focusing on more straightforward mixed-methods designs, with the option to explore variations as needed. In this book, we present three fundamental mixed-methods designs—convergent, explanatory sequential, and exploratory sequential—along with one advanced design, the embedded intervention, all accompanied by examples of their application in health research.

These basic designs provide a solid foundation for researchers, while the embedded intervention design adds complexity and depth for more advanced studies. By adopting these designs, researchers can ensure methodological clarity and adaptability, particularly in the field of health research, where the integration of qualitative and quantitative data can lead to richer, more actionable insights.

4.4.1 Convergent Design

The convergent design is one of the most well-known and widely used approaches in mixed-methods research. Jick [5] highlighted the use of triangulation, and it remains one of the most common methods employed across various disciplines. Initially, the convergent design was conceived as a triangulation design, where two different methods—qualitative and quantitative—were used to gather complementary results on the same topic. However, it is often confused with the concept of triangulation in purely qualitative research, and researchers frequently use this design for purposes beyond triangulated findings.

Since its inception, this design has been referred to by several different names, including

Fig. 4.2 Convergent
design

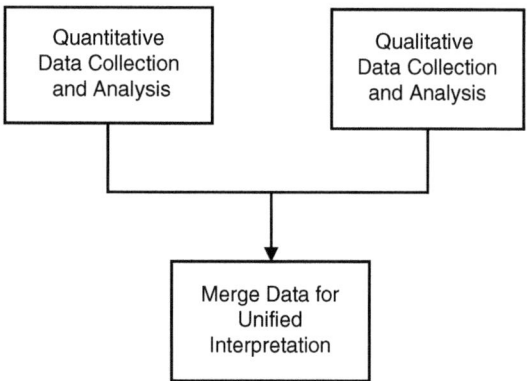

simultaneous triangulation [6], parallel study [7], convergence model [8], and concurrent triangulation [9]. Despite the various terms, the core principle remains the same: in a convergent design, the researcher collects and analyses both quantitative and qualitative data during the same phase of the research process, then merges the two sets of results into a unified interpretation (Fig. 4.2).

In a convergent design, both quantitative and qualitative data are collected simultaneously but analyzed separately, with the findings of one phase not reliant on the results of the other [10]. Typically, this design assigns equal importance to both quantitative and qualitative data, and the results are integrated during the interpretation phase, where meta-inferences are drawn.

One of the main advantages of this approach is its efficiency—since all data are collected concurrently, the study population remains accessible throughout the process. This is especially valuable in fields like nursing and healthcare, where patients may be discharged, making follow-up recruitment challenging. However, a key challenge arises when the findings do not converge as expected, but rather diverge. Novice researchers often hope for convergence to neatly tie up their results and enhance the validity of their findings. It is important to note, as Skamagki et al. [4] discuss, that divergence in findings does not necessarily indicate a problem with the study and can instead offer valuable insights into the complexity of the research topic.

An example of a study utilizing this design examined the impact of a new patient-centered care model in a hospital setting. Quantitative data were collected from 100 patients through a structured survey assessing their satisfaction with care, while qualitative data were gathered through in-depth interviews with 15 healthcare providers to explore their experiences and perspectives on the implementation of the new model. The simultaneous collection of both datasets allowed researchers to analyze patient outcomes alongside provider insights. This combination provided a more comprehensive understanding of the effectiveness of the care model, with the qualitative data offering contextual details that enriched the quantitative findings. The convergence of the two data sets revealed a strong alignment between patient satisfaction and provider support for the model, reinforcing the overall validity of the study.

4.5   Explanatory Sequential Design

The explanatory sequential design typically involves a dominant quantitative phase, followed by a smaller, complementary qualitative phase, aimed at elaborating on and clarifying the quantitative findings Fig. 4.3. Data collection and analysis proceed in a sequential manner, with the results from the quantitative phase shaping the

Fig. 4.3 Explanatory
sequential design

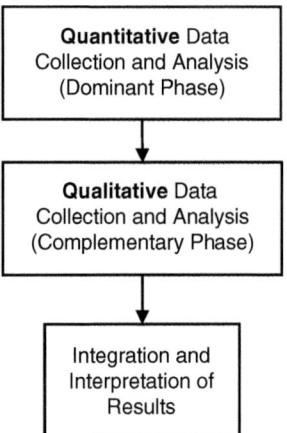

structure and focus of the subsequent qualitative phase. This design is particularly valuable when a researcher aims to identify trends and relationships using quantitative data while also seeking to understand the underlying mechanisms or reasons driving those patterns. It allows for the integration of numerical analysis with qualitative insights, providing a more comprehensive explanation of the observed trends. By combining both approaches, researchers can not only quantify relationships but also explore the contextual factors and motivations behind the data, leading to a deeper and more holistic understanding of the research findings.

Given the dominance of the quantitative phase, this design is particularly useful when qualitative insights are needed to explain significant or nonsignificant quantitative outcomes, highlight high-performing cases, examine outliers, or explore unexpected findings in greater depth. Additionally, the explanatory design is valuable when the researcher intends to form groups based on quantitative outcomes and conduct qualitative follow-up studies with those groups. It can also be used to inform purposeful sampling for qualitative research by utilizing quantitative participant characteristics. This method allows for a more nuanced understanding of the data by integrating statistical results with rich, detailed narratives.

The explanatory design is a straightforward mixed-methods approach, appealing to quantitative researchers by starting with a strong quantitative phase. Its two-phase structure allows data collection and analysis in separate stages, making it manageable for individual researchers without the need for a large team. The clear organization of quantitative and qualitative sections simplifies report writing and ensures easy reader comprehension. Additionally, the flexibility to adapt the qualitative phase based on initial quantitative results adds to its versatility, offering a balance between quantitative rigor and qualitative depth.

While the explanatory design is straightforward, researchers must anticipate certain challenges. It requires significant time, as the qualitative phase often takes longer than the quantitative phase, even with fewer participants. One key challenge is that, since this design is emergent and the second phase cannot be fully developed until the first phase is completed, the study may need to go before an ethics committee or institutional review board (IRB) a second time to gain approval for the qualitative phase. Researchers can mitigate this by outlining a tentative plan and informing participants of potential follow-up. Additionally, determining which quantitative results to explore further and deciding participant selection criteria, such as demographics or key predictors, are essential.

Addressing these challenges early can help ensure smooth implementation.

For example, an explanatory sequential design was utilized to explore the impact of nurse burnout on patient care quality within a busy hospital setting. In the initial phase, surveys were distributed to nursing staff to assess burnout levels and identify contributing factors such as workload, emotional exhaustion, and job satisfaction. Based on the survey findings, a sub-group of nurses experiencing high burnout was selected for qualitative interviews. These interviews offered in-depth insights into how burnout influenced their ability to deliver quality patient care and affected their personal well-being. This mixed-methods approach provided a comprehensive understanding of both the quantitative patterns and the personal experiences of nurse burnout in the hospital context.

4.6   Exploratory Sequential Design

The exploratory sequential design is defined by its initial qualitative phase, which transitions into a quantitative phase. This design is particularly valuable when developing instruments where none exist, identifying previously unknown variables, or formulating new theories or hypotheses. The subsequent quantitative phase is used to test the developed instrument or

to generalize the qualitative findings to a broader population (Fig. 4.4). The priority between the qualitative and quantitative phases depends on the study's goals: if the focus is on theory development, the qualitative phase typically dominates, while in cases of instrument development and testing, the quantitative phase often takes precedence.

The primary purpose of the exploratory design is to generalize qualitative findings from a small group in the initial phase to a larger sample in the subsequent quantitative phase. Similar to the explanatory design, the two-phase structure ensures that insights gained from the first, qualitative phase inform or shape the second, quantitative phase. This design is particularly useful when exploration is necessary due to the lack of available instruments, unknown variables, or the absence of a guiding framework or theory. Since it begins with a qualitative approach, the design is ideal for in-depth exploration of a phenomenon. It is especially valuable for researchers who need to develop and test new instruments or identify key variables for quantitative analysis. Additionally, it works well when the goal is to generalize qualitative findings to larger populations, test aspects of an emerging theory, or measure the prevalence and dimensions of a phenomenon. This approach allows for both detailed exploration and broader validation, offering a comprehensive understanding of the research topic.

Fig. 4.4 Exploratory sequential design

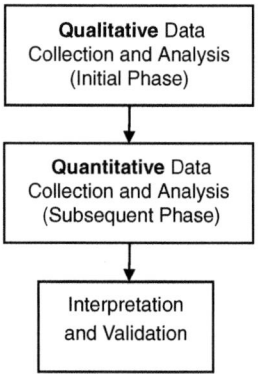

Qualitative data is collected first to explore a phenomenon, followed by quantitative data to generalize findings or test instruments.

The exploratory design shares many of the same advantages and challenges as the explanatory design, such as the two-phase structure and the need for careful planning. However, a unique challenge in the exploratory design lies in the added complexity of developing and testing a new instrument, which can be time-consuming and require additional steps to ensure its validity and reliability. This aspect of instrument creation introduces an extra layer of difficulty, making the exploratory process more demanding compared to the explanatory design.

For example, Dehghani [11] conducted a sequential exploratory study was conducted to develop and validate a clinical judgment capability questionnaire for nurses. In the first phase, qualitative interviews were carried out with 12 experienced clinical nurses to explore the dimensions of clinical judgment in their daily practice. This resulted in the identification of key elements of clinical judgment, such as noticing, interpreting, responding, and reflecting. These findings were then used to design a 22-item questionnaire. In the second phase, this newly developed questionnaire was administered to 181 nurses to assess its validity and reliability. The results provided valuable insights into the clinical judgment capabilities of nurses and helped to refine the tool for broader use in clinical settings. This approach allowed researchers to create a robust and culturally relevant instrument for measuring clinical judgment in nursing, which can now be used to evaluate and improve nursing education and practice.

4.7 Embedded Design

The embedded design is a mixed-methods approach where the researcher integrates both quantitative and qualitative data collection and analysis within a traditional research framework either predominantly quantitative or qualitative. The second data set can be collected and analyzed before, during, or after the primary data collection phase of the larger design. In some cases, one data set plays a secondary, supportive role (Fig. 4.5). For instance, a qualitative component might be embedded within a quantitative experiment to provide additional insights. In other scenarios, both quantitative and qualitative approaches are embedded into a single traditional design, such as a mixed-methods case study, where both types of data are used to explore a case. Additionally, researchers can integrate quantitative and qualitative methods into specific procedures, like social network analysis, to enhance the depth and breadth of the study's find-

Fig. 4.5 Embedded design

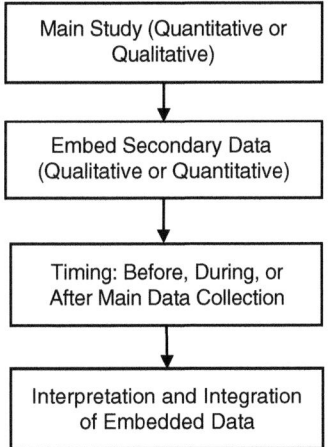

Main Study (Quantitative or Qualitative)

Embed Secondary Data (Qualitative or Quantitative)

Timing: Before, During, or After Main Data Collection

Interpretation and Integration of Embedded Data

Embedded Design integrates secondary qualitative or quantitative data within a primary study to enhance insights and understanding.

ings. This flexibility allows for a richer understanding of complex research questions.

The rationale behind this design is that a single data set may be insufficient to address all research questions, and different types of questions require distinct data types. In an embedded experimental mixed-methods design, researchers employ this approach when qualitative data is necessary to answer a secondary research question within a predominantly quantitative study. For example, qualitative data may be embedded to enhance recruitment processes, examine the implementation of an intervention, or understand participants' reactions to the experiment. Importantly, the purpose of collecting qualitative data is connected to, but distinct from, the primary goal of the experiment, which is to determine if the treatment has a significant effect. This sets the embedded design apart from the convergent design, where both qualitative and quantitative methods are used to address a single overarching research question. The embedded approach allows for a more nuanced exploration of secondary aspects that complement the main inquiry.

The embedded design has several strengths. It is ideal when time or resources are limited, as one data type is prioritized, reducing the need for extensive data collection. Adding supplemental data enhances the overall study design. Since different methods address distinct research questions, it works well in team settings, allowing members to focus on their expertise. Additionally, the results can be published separately, providing flexibility. This design may also appeal to funding agencies familiar with traditional research, as it maintains a primary focus on one method while incorporating mixed methods.

The embedded design comes with several challenges that require careful planning. Researchers must have expertise in both the primary quantitative or qualitative design and mixed methods. It is important to clearly define the primary and secondary objectives for collecting qualitative (or quantitative) data within the larger study. Another challenge is deciding when to collect qualitative data—before, during, or after the intervention—based on its purpose, such as shaping the intervention or explaining results. Integrating the results can be difficult when the methods address different research questions, but unlike the convergent design, merging data sets is not necessary, and they can be reported separately. Additionally, collecting qualitative data during the intervention risks introducing bias that may affect the experiment's outcomes.

Alilyyani et al. [12] conducted an embedded mixed-methods study to examine the leadership skills of nursing staff and intern nursing students. The study primarily used quantitative data from a survey assessing leadership capabilities, while qualitative data was embedded to explore participants' experiences and perceptions in greater depth. The qualitative data, collected through open-ended questions, provided additional insights into strategies for enhancing leadership skills and the obstacles nurses face in their development. By embedding qualitative data within a largely quantitative framework, the study offered a more comprehensive understanding of how experience and education impact leadership abilities in nursing professionals.

4.8   Critical Challenges in Mixed-Methods Research

Key challenges in mixed-methods research have garnered attention, particularly concerning data analysis, and integration of findings. These challenges are pivotal as they directly influence the robustness of conclusions and the overall validity of the research outcomes.

4.8.1   Data Analysis

In most mixed-methods studies, quantitative and qualitative data are usually analyzed independently, with each adhering to the analytical methods relevant to its own tradition. The combination of results typically takes place during the interpretation phase. However, there is great potential to improve the integration of data analysis in mixed-methods research by utilizing a variety of innovative techniques. Progress in these integrated approaches can deepen the insights derived, providing a more comprehensive understanding of the research issue. In this section, two key aspects will be discussed: typology development and data transformation, both of which are critical to advancing data analysis in mixed-methods research.

4.8.1.1 Typology Development

The analysis from one method often forms the basis for analyzing the other, with quantitative data frequently providing a structure upon which qualitative data are aligned. A coding matrix is typically created, where the main quantitative findings are highlighted, followed by a section for the corresponding qualitative data to explain those findings. Afterward, the qualitative data usually undergo further thematic analysis. This approach proves especially beneficial in sequential explanatory designs, as it ensures that questions arising from the quantitative phase are addressed. However, it is equally essential not to overlook other qualitative insights, even if they do not directly correlate with the quantitative findings, as they may offer additional valuable perspectives.

For example, begin by conducting a quantitative survey and perform factor analysis to identify key factors. These factors can then serve as a framework, or typology, for guiding the identification of themes in qualitative data, such as those emerging from interviews and observations. This process allows for a structured approach to integrating data, enhancing the ability to draw meaningful connections between the quantitative and qualitative findings, while also providing a more nuanced understanding of the research problem.

4.8.1.2 Data Transformation

Data transformation in mixed-methods research involves converting one form of data into another. One approach is qualitizing data, where quantitative data are transformed into qualitative narratives. Although this method is less common, it often involves constructing detailed narrative profiles from the numerical data.

More frequently, quantitizing occurs, where qualitative data are converted into quantitative

forms. This can be achieved by assigning numerical or binary values to qualitative data, followed by statistical analysis (). For instance, participants' responses to interview questions may be "counted," producing descriptive statistics that reveal patterns that might have been overlooked through qualitative analysis alone ().

Quantitizing can add depth to mixed-methods studies by allowing patterns in qualitative data to be analyzed statistically; however, caution is necessary. Qualitative data are inherently non-random and not typically normally distributed, which can affect the accuracy of statistical tests and limit the generalizability of the results (). Furthermore, over-reliance on quantitizing risks diminishing the richness and depth of qualitative data. Therefore, it is important to use this method as a complement to, rather than a replacement for, traditional qualitative analysis.

4.8.2   Integration

Data integration has emerged as a central focus in mixed-methods research and is one of the key challenges for researchers using these designs. Much of the existing literature discusses integration as the blending of qualitative and quantitative data, but it encompasses more than that. Integration refers to the merging of both the quantitative and qualitative components throughout a study, representing the points at which the different phases intersect. This process is fundamental to the "mixing" that defines a mixed-methods approach. Some researchers argue that readers of mixed-methods studies deserve more than just parallel accounts of findings that fail to connect meaningfully. Effective integration should create a synergistic outcome, where the combination of methods offers insights that exceed the sum of their individual parts.

Moving beyond the idea that integration is limited to data alone, scholars have identified how integration can occur across multiple levels: in the design, the methods, and the reporting/interpretation stages of the research. A well-integrated mixed-methods study not only enhances the depth of understanding but also ensures that the strengths of both qualitative and quantitative approaches are fully realized throughout the research process.

4.8.2.1 Integration at the Methods Level

At the methods level, integration can occur at multiple stages, particularly in studies employing a sequential design. For instance, findings from the initial phase may guide the development of a sampling frame for the subsequent phase. This is common in explanatory designs, where a purposive sample is selected in the qualitative phase to further explore unusual or unexpected results from the quantitative phase. Another form of integration occurs when the outcomes of the first phase directly influence the design of the second, a process referred to as "building" by Hall and Mansfield [13].

In exploratory designs, qualitative findings from interviews in the first phase may be used to create a survey or instrument that is later tested quantitatively in the second phase. Conversely, in explanatory designs, quantitative results from the first phase can shape the development of interview guides or other tools, such as vignettes, for use in the qualitative phase. This helps to ensure that specific issues or patterns identified earlier are fully explored. Finally, integration at the methods level also occurs during data analysis, where the interplay between qualitative and quantitative data allows for a more comprehensive understanding, as previously discussed.

Incorporating integration at these various stages ensures a more cohesive research process, allowing each phase to build on and inform the next, ultimately contributing to richer, more meaningful results.

4.8.2.2 Integration at the Reporting/ Interpretation Level

In many mixed-methods studies, findings are often presented separately; however, there is a growing emphasis on increasing the integration of data within the findings section. One effective approach is to present quantitative and qualitative results together, organized according to themes. This method of thematic integration is particu-

larly valuable in convergent designs, where overarching meta-themes are developed from both data sources. For studies that present findings separately, integration can still be achieved through a "weaving" technique, where quantitative results are briefly interwoven with qualitative insights to act as anchors for deeper explanations. This strategy works well in explanatory designs, where quantitative and qualitative findings are largely presented independently, but key quantitative results are incorporated into the qualitative narrative to help provide context or "hooks" for the explanatory phase.

Another useful strategy for enhancing integration is the use of joint displays. For instance, in sequential explanatory studies, joint displays might involve creating a table with separate columns for quantitative and qualitative findings. A third column can then be added to demonstrate how the qualitative data explain or expand on the quantitative results. This method allows for a clear visual representation of how both sets of data are linked, facilitating a deeper interpretation of the findings.

Utilizing these integration techniques enables researchers to craft a more cohesive and comprehensive narrative, providing readers with a clearer understanding of how both types of data contribute to the overall conclusions.

4.8.2.3 Integration at the Discussion Level

At a minimum, integration in a mixed-methods study must occur within the discussion section. In this part of the study, conclusions may initially be drawn from the quantitative and qualitative phases independently. However, a critical step is the development of meta-inferences, which are comprehensive conclusions derived from the combination of both quantitative and qualitative data. Meta-inferences extend beyond the insights gained from each component in isolation, offering a more complete and unified understanding of the research findings. These integrative conclusions should effectively address the core questions posed in the mixed-methods design.

In addition to synthesizing the findings, the discussion should explore how the integration of data has enriched the overall interpretation, highlighting any novel insights or patterns that emerged only through the blending of both approaches. This level of integration ultimately strengthens the research by providing a deeper, more holistic answer to the study's research questions.

4.9 Validity in Mixed Method

Although mixed-methods research has gained widespread use, the issue of validity associated with such designs remains a topic of debate [14]. This challenge has been recognized by many mixed-methods researchers, with Onwuegbuzie and Johnson [15] acknowledging that the blending of the unique strengths and distinct shortcomings of both qualitative and quantitative methods makes it difficult to evaluate the validity of mixed-methods research. Designing mixed-methods research involves managing numerous primary and secondary characteristics that require careful attention. It is essential that the study design aligns with the research questions or objectives [3, 16].

The design should follow either a concurrent or sequential approach to accurately capture the phenomenon being investigated. In a concurrent design, both qualitative and quantitative components are carried out simultaneously, while in a sequential design, one component follows the other, with either the quantitative phase preceding the qualitative or vice versa [17]. A notable challenge within mixed-methods research, as observed by Creswell and Plano Clark [10], is the variety of terms used to describe different mixed-methods designs, leading to confusion in terminology. However, they believe that as the field of mixed-methods research continues to evolve, this issue will gradually improve.

For the purpose of ensuring validity, the design of a mixed-methods study must be transparent and address all aspects related to credibility and trustworthiness, as highlighted by leading scholars in the field [15, 18]. A robust design should embody the following key characteristics, as outlined by these researchers:

Suitability: This refers to the alignment of the study's approaches with its research question(s). The design must be appropriate and relevant to effectively answer the research question, ensuring that the methodology is in harmony with the study's objectives.

Analytical Adequacy: This focuses on whether the data analysis methods are rigorous and appropriate for addressing the research question(s). It ensures that the chosen analytical techniques are capable of accurately interpreting the data.

Integrative Efficacy: This assesses whether the meta-inferences adequately integrate findings from both the quantitative and qualitative components of the study. Successful integration allows for a comprehensive understanding of the research problem by combining insights from both methodological approaches.

Inference Transferability: This refers to the generalizability of the findings from both the quantitative and qualitative aspects of the study. Transferability is examined across multiple dimensions, including population transferability (applying results to different individuals or groups), ecological transferability (applicability to various contexts or environments), and operational transferability (adaptation of results to different methods of evaluating behaviors).

Since mixed-methods design involves the collection, analysis, and integration of both qualitative and quantitative data within a single or multi-phase study [19], it requires a combination of non-numerical and numerical data. Qualitative data are typically collected through unstructured questionnaires, while quantitative data are gathered using structured questionnaires. The integration of these data can occur in three main ways [10]: concurrent mixed analysis, where both qualitative and quantitative data are analyzed simultaneously; sequential qualitative–quantitative analysis, where qualitative data are analyzed first, followed by quantitative data; and sequential quantitative-qualitative analysis, where the quantitative analysis is conducted first, followed by qualitative analysis [20].

It is important to recognize that qualitative and quantitative methods, as distinct approaches, each have their *own validation techniques*. In quantitative research, validity refers to the accuracy of measurement, and reliability refers to the consistency of results, together forming the foundation of rigor. In qualitative research, rigor is maintained through specific quality criteria established by experts in the field.

Therefore, the integration of both qualitative and quantitative methods in mixed-methods research not only enhances the richness of the data but also requires careful attention to the distinct ways in which validity and reliability are addressed in each approach to ensure the overall credibility of the study.

References

1. Doyle L, Brady A-M, Byrne G. An overview of mixed methods research—revisited. J Res Nurs. 2016;21:623–35. https://doi.org/10.1177/1744987116674257.
2. Creswell JW, Creswell JD. Research design: qualitative, quantitative, and mixed methods approaches. Thousand Oaks: SAGE; 2023.
3. Bazeley P. Conceptualizing integration in mixed methods research. J Mixed Methods Res. 2024;18:225–34. https://doi.org/10.1177/15586898241253636.
4. Skamagki G, King A, Carpenter C, Wåhlin C. The concept of integration in mixed methods research: a step-by-step guide using an example study in physiotherapy. Physiother Theory Pract. 2024;40:197–204. https://doi.org/10.1080/09593985.2022.2120375.
5. Jick TD. Mixing qualitative and quantitative methods: triangulation in action. Adm Sci Q. 1979;24:602–11. https://doi.org/10.2307/2392366.
6. Morse JM. Approaches to qualitative-quantitative methodological triangulation. Nurs Res. 1991;40:120.
7. Tashakkori A, Teddlie C. SAGE handbook of mixed methods in social & behavioral research. Thousand Oaks: SAGE; 2021.
8. Creswell JW. Mixed-method research: introduction and application. In: Cizek GJ, editor. Handbook of educational policy. San Diego: Academic Press; 1999. p. 455–72.
9. Creswell J, Clark V, Gutmann M, Hanson W. Advance mixed methods research designs. In: Handbook of mixed methods in social and behavioral research. Thousand Oaks: SAGE; 2003. p. 209–40.
10. Creswell JW, Plano Clark VL. Mapping design trends and evolving directions using the Sage handbook of mixed methods research design. In: Poth CN, editor. The Sage handbook of mixed methods research design. Thousand Oaks: SAGE; 2023.
11. Dehghani A. Development and validation of the clinical judgment capability questionnaire in nurses: a sequential exploratory mixed method study. Int J Nurs Stud Adv. 2024;6:100191. https://doi.org/10.1016/j.ijnsa.2024.100191.
12. Alilyyani B, Althobaiti E, Al-Talhi M, et al. Nursing experience and leadership skills among staff nurses and intern nursing students in Saudi Arabia: a mixed methods study. BMC Nurs. 2024;23:87. https://doi.org/10.1186/s12912-024-01750-1.
13. Hall J, Mansfield L. The benefits and complexities of integrating mixed method findings using the pillar integration process: a workplace health intervention case study. Journal of Mixed Methods Research. SAGE Publications; 2023. Aug 17;15586898231196287.
14. Adu J, Owusu MF, Martin-Yeboah E, et al. A discussion of some controversies in mixed methods research for emerging researchers. Methodol Innov. 2022;15:321–30. https://doi.org/10.1177/20597991221123398.
15. Onwuegbuzie AJ, Johnson RB. The validity issue in mixed research. Res Sch. 2006;13:48–63.
16. Johnson RE, Grove AL, Clarke A. Pillar integration process: a joint display technique to integrate data in mixed methods research. J Mixed Methods Res. 2019;13:301–20. https://doi.org/10.1177/1558689817743108.
17. Johnson RB. Dialectical pluralism and integration in mixed methods research. In: Philosophical foundations of mixed methods research. Milton Park: Routledge; 2023.
18. Tashakkori A, Teddlie C. Quality of inferences in mixed methods research: calling for an integrative framework. In: Bergman MM, editor. Advances in mixed methods research: theories and applications. London: SAGE; 2008.
19. Guetterman TC, Manojlovich M. Grand rounds in methodology: designing for integration in mixed methods research. BMJ Qual Saf. 2024;33:470–8. https://doi.org/10.1136/bmjqs-2023-016112.
20. Fàbregues S, Escalante-Barrios EL, Turk ST, et al. Assessing quality in mixed methods research: concepts, frameworks, and criteria. In: Cameron R, Golenko X, editors. Handbook of mixed methods research in business and management. Cheltenham: Edward Elgar; 2023. p. 76–93.

Ethics in Nursing Research

5

Learning Outcomes

By the end of this chapter, readers should be able to:

1. Understand the historical context of unethical research practices and their impact on current ethical guidelines.
2. Explain the ethical principles of beneficence, respect for human dignity, and justice as they apply to nursing research.
3. Describe the importance of informed consent and how it protects participants in research studies.
4. Identify the unique ethical challenges involved in conducting research with vulnerable populations.
5. Evaluate the role of Institutional Review Boards (IRBs) in safeguarding the rights and welfare of research participants.

5.1 Introduction

In nursing research, the same ethical standards that apply to all research involving human participants must be rigorously followed. Nurses are responsible not only for understanding and applying these ethical principles in their own research but also for critically evaluating and reviewing the research of others. Ethical concerns permeate every aspect of both the design and execution of a study. Therefore, before discussing research design techniques, it is essential to consider the major ethical principles involved in developing research plans.

Health research is generally undertaken to improve healthcare delivery and develop new treatments or interventions. Nursing research, in particular, emphasizes the multifaceted roles that nurses play in healthcare, aiming to benefit patients and enhance their experiences and outcomes. However, as the line between nursing practice and research data collection becomes increasingly blurred, ethical concerns in nursing research have become more pronounced. The growing volume of research has amplified concerns about protecting the rights of study participants, especially in nursing, where the distinction between expected practice and research can often be unclear.

Ethical challenges are particularly complex for nurse researchers because ethical requirements may at times seem to conflict with the need to produce the highest quality evidence for practice. Nevertheless, ethical approval must always be secured before initiating any research involving human participants, and nurse researchers must also ensure their professional conduct aligns with national codes of practice. The balance between maintaining ethical integrity and producing robust evidence is critical, ensuring that the rights and well-being of participants are safeguarded while advancing healthcare knowledge.

Human participants are frequently involved in research, particularly in nursing studies, making it crucial to ensure their rights are fully protected. Although the necessity of ethical conduct may seem obvious, history has shown that ethical considerations have not always been given the attention they deserve. In several cases, participants' rights and well-being were compromised, underscoring the importance of clear ethical standards.

This chapter explores the reasons ethical guidelines have become a fundamental part of research involving human participants. As research expanded, the protection of dignity, rights, and safety became increasingly critical, prompting the development of ethical frameworks that researchers, including those in nursing, must follow. These guidelines play an essential role in ensuring that participants' rights are upheld, even as the field continues to advance knowledge and improve healthcare outcomes.

5.2   Historical Overview of Unethical Research

The twentieth century marked a significant rise in research involving human subjects, leading to numerous groundbreaking medical advancements. However, formal ethical guidelines and standards were not introduced until the early twentieth century, highlighting the urgent need for oversight and regulation to safeguard human participants. Several well-known studies from this period serve as important historical examples. Some studies resulted in positive outcomes, but others exposed serious ethical failings. These events underscored the necessity for more robust ethical standards to ensure the protection and well-being of the public in future research.

The twentieth century witnessed a dramatic rise in human subject research, leading to significant medical advancements. However, formal ethical guidelines and standards were only introduced later in the early twentieth century, making it clear that rigorous ethical oversight was urgently needed to protect human participants. Several renowned research studies from this

period have shaped the historical understanding of ethical considerations in research. Some produced valuable outcomes, yet others revealed serious ethical failings. These events underscored the critical need for stricter ethical standards to safeguard public welfare.

The recognition of the necessity for regulated ethical constraints emerged as a result of numerous egregious instances of unethical practices during the twentieth century. Four experimental studies are particularly notorious for their unethical treatment of human participants: the Nazi medical experiments, the Tuskegee Syphilis Study, and the Willowbrook Study. Nurses played a role in carrying out these studies, although the primary researchers were physicians. These unethical experiments underscore the vital importance of ethical conduct for nurses, whether they are reviewing or directly participating in research. These cases also played a significant role in shaping the ethical codes and regulations that continue to guide modern research practices today.

5.2.1   Nazi Medical Experiments (1939–1945)

During World War II, the Nazi regime conducted horrific and unethical medical experiments on prisoners, particularly those held in concentration camps. These experiments were carried out without consent and targeted individuals deemed "worthless" by the regime, including Jews and prisoners of war. Participants were subjected to extreme conditions, such as exposure to high altitudes, freezing temperatures, poisons, and infections, as well as undergoing surgeries without anesthesia. The experiments resulted in immense suffering, permanent harm, and often death, violating the fundamental rights of the subjects through unjust selection and forced participation. Beyond their extreme cruelty, these studies were poorly designed and yielded little, if any, scientific value. These atrocities serve as a stark reminder of the essential need for stringent ethical standards in research to protect human dignity and prevent the exploitation of vulnerable populations.

5.2.2   Tuskegee Syphilis Study (1932–1972)

The Tuskegee Syphilis Study, initiated by the U.S. Public Health Service in 1932, is a notorious case of unethical medical research. Involving 600 African American men from Tuskegee, Alabama, the study misled participants about its true purpose, claiming to treat "bad blood" while actually observing the natural progression of untreated syphilis. Despite penicillin being identified as an effective treatment in the 1940s, the men were deliberately denied care, leading to preventable deaths and suffering.

Even after published reports in the 1930s and 1969, the study continued until public outrage, sparked by a 1972 Washington Star article, forced its termination. Investigations revealed the gross ethical violations. This study remains a stark reminder of the need for strict ethical standards and protections for vulnerable populations in research.

5.2.3   Willowbrook Hepatitis Study (1956–1972)

Dr. Saul Krugman conducted a controversial study at Willowbrook State School in Staten Island, New York, where children with intellectual disabilities were deliberately infected with hepatitis to study the disease's progression and test treatments. Researchers justified their actions by claiming that hepatitis was already prevalent in the institution, but critics condemned the unethical use of vulnerable children. Parents were often coerced into consenting, being told that participation would secure better care for their children. In 1966, Henry Beecher highlighted the Willowbrook Study in the New England Journal of Medicine as a prime example of unethical research. Despite attempts to defend the study, it faced widespread criticism for its exploitative nature and lack of informed consent. The study is now considered a significant violation of medical ethics, highlighting the need for stronger protections for vulnerable populations in research.

5.3   Ethical Standards in Nursing Research

Researchers working with human participants often face complex ethical challenges, balancing the need to advance knowledge and produce high-quality evidence with the obligation to safeguard human rights. This is particularly true for nurse researchers, whose roles as caregivers may at times conflict with their responsibilities as researchers, such as when they feel compelled to provide immediate care at the expense of strictly following research protocols. These dilemmas underscore the critical importance of ethical codes, which guide researchers in managing their dual responsibilities while maintaining professional integrity.

The development of these ethical frameworks was largely driven by the history of unethical research practices, most notably highlighted by the Nuremberg Trials, which revealed the horrific Nazi war crimes. The trials led to the creation of the Nuremberg Code in 1947, a landmark document that established the principle of voluntary, informed consent and set the standard for ethical research involving human subjects [1]. This code became the foundation for international ethical standards and laws that aim to protect participants' rights and ensure researchers are held accountable.

The Nuremberg Code laid the groundwork for the creation of the Declaration of Helsinki, which was first adopted in 1964 [2]. One of the key aspects of the Declaration was distinguishing between therapeutic and non-therapeutic research. Therapeutic research offers participants the chance to receive experimental treatments that could potentially benefit their health. In contrast, non-therapeutic research is conducted to advance scientific knowledge, with no direct benefit expected for the participants involved, though future patients may ultimately gain from the findings. Researchers are tasked with safeguarding the health, privacy, and dignity of participants, while carefully selecting study topics that balance the risks and burdens for those involved. The World Medical Association (WMA) continues to play a pivotal role in refining these ethical standards, with the most recent revision of the Declaration published in 2013 [3]. These revisions ensure that research practices evolve alongside advancements in medicine, maintaining a focus on ethical responsibility.

The formal consideration of research ethics in nursing began to develop in the 1950s. During this period, the primary focus was on fundamental values, emphasizing the responsibility of researchers to uphold what is morally right and beneficial [4]. In 1953, the International Council of Nurses (ICN) introduced the Code of Ethics for Nurses, which served as a foundation for nursing associations in various countries to establish their own ethical standards of practice. This milestone not only shaped the ethical conduct of nurses but also laid the groundwork for the ethical frameworks that would guide nursing research in the future, ensuring that nurses maintain accountability and integrity in both clinical and research settings.

The discussion of research ethics specific to nursing began to take shape in the 1950s, with a focus on fundamental principles related to researchers' responsibilities to act in ways that promote good and uphold moral integrity. In 1953, the International Council of Nurses (ICN) introduced the Code of Ethics for Nurses, which became the foundation for nursing associations worldwide to establish their own ethical standards [5]. Since its initial adoption, the ICN Code has undergone several revisions, with the most recent update occurring in 2021, ensuring it remains relevant and aligned with contemporary nursing practices and ethical challenges [6].

The Belmont Report, published in 1979 by the [7], marked a significant milestone in establishing ethical guidelines for research. At the heart of the Belmont Report are three core ethical principles: beneficence, respect for human dignity, and justice. These principles form the foundation for ethical research standards, ensuring that studies prioritize the well-being of participants, respect their autonomy, and promote fairness in the selection and treatment of subjects. Additionally, the report distinguished between therapeutic and non-therapeutic research, providing clarity on

how research findings should be applied in medical practice.

The evolution of these ethical guidelines has been essential not only for preventing future abuses but also for building trust between researchers and the public. Establishing clear protocols and prioritizing the dignity and safety of participants, these codes have shaped modern research ethics, ensuring that scientific progress is pursued responsibly and ethically.

5.4   Ethical Principle in Research

Protecting research participants goes beyond merely complying with laws and standards; it requires researchers to be guided by fundamental ethical principles that safeguard the rights and dignity of individuals. Historical cases of unethical research highlight the critical need for such protections. Three core principles form the foundation of ethical research: **beneficence, respect for persons** and **justice**. Respect for persons involves treating individuals as autonomous agents, securing informed consent, and allowing them the freedom to withdraw from the study. Vulnerable populations, such as children, individuals with illnesses, and prisoners, require additional safeguards. These ethical principles not only protect participants' rights but also promote integrity among nurses, research partners, and institutions. Furthermore, they ensure the validity and reliability of research, fostering trust and accountability in nursing studies. Upholding these principles enables nursing research to maintain high ethical standards while responsibly advancing knowledge.

5.4.1   Beneficence

Beneficence, the principle of doing good, places a responsibility on researchers to minimize harm and maximize benefits. Research involving human subjects should aim to provide benefits, either directly to the participants or, more commonly, to others. This principle covers several aspects, including the obligation to promote participants' welfare and safeguard their well-being. Research should not only strive to benefit individual participants but also contribute positively to society. To uphold this principle, researchers must conduct a thorough risk–benefit analysis, carefully weighing potential and perceived risks against anticipated benefits. Additionally, ongoing monitoring throughout the study is crucial to continuously assess and balance these risks and benefits, ensuring that participant welfare remains a priority at every stage.

5.4.2 Freedom from Harm and Discomfort

Researchers have a duty to avoid, prevent, or minimize harm, a principle known as *nonmaleficence (do no harm)*, in studies involving human participants. It is essential that participants are not exposed to unnecessary risks of harm or discomfort, and their involvement must be crucial to achieving important scientific and societal goals that cannot be attained by other means. In human research, harm and discomfort can take various forms, including physical (such as injury or fatigue), emotional (such as stress or fear), social (such as loss of social support), financial (such as loss of wages), or cognitive (such as confusion or mental exhaustion). Ethical researchers must implement measures to reduce all types of harm and discomfort, even if temporary. Furthermore, ensuring that participants are fully informed about potential risks and providing support throughout the study are key components of ethical responsibility.

Research should be conducted by qualified individuals, particularly when using hazardous equipment or procedures. Ethical researchers must be ready to halt a study if it risks injury, death, or distress. Testing new medical procedures should typically begin with animals or tissue cultures before involving humans. While protecting against physical harm is straightforward, psychological impacts require careful attention. Personal questions may reveal sensitive information, and researchers must consider emotional effects. This is especially crucial in **quali-**

tative research, where deep probing may uncover repressed fears. Researchers must be vigilant about these risks and provide appropriate support or referrals for participants who experience emotional distress during or after the study.

5.4.2.1 Protection from Exploitation

Participants in a study should not be placed at a disadvantage or exposed to harm as a result of their involvement. They must be assured that their participation, and any information they provide, will not be used against them in any way. For instance, individuals sharing details about their mental health history should not fear discrimination in future employment, and those disclosing sensitive personal relationships should not worry about this information being used to harm their reputation. Ensuring that participants fully understand the protections in place, including **confidentiality** and **data privacy** measures, is critical to building trust and safeguarding their rights throughout the research process.

Study participants form a unique relationship with researchers, and it's crucial that this relationship is not exploited. Exploitation can be overt, like sexual misconduct or using donated blood for commercial purposes but can also be subtle. For example, if participants consent to a single interview and the researcher later uses their data for a different study without additional consent, it can breach their trust. Nurse researchers must be cautious, as patients may agree out of loyalty to the nurse-patient relationship, not fully grasping the research implications.

In qualitative research, emotional distance often decreases over time, sometimes creating a pseudo therapeutic relationship, which increases the risk of unintentional exploitation [8]. However, qualitative researchers can also do more good because of the relationships they form with participants. Qualitative nurse researchers should prioritize the therapeutic needs of nursing over research goals if any conflicts arise [9]. Furthermore, researchers should clearly communicate the boundaries of their role from the outset, ensuring participants understand both the research and clinical dimensions to prevent any misunderstanding or potential exploitation.

5.4.3 Respect for Human Dignity

The principle of respect for human dignity is a fundamental ethical guideline that emphasizes treating individuals with autonomy and respect. It encompasses two fundamental rights: the right to self-determination, allowing individuals to make their own informed decisions, and the right to full disclosure, ensuring that all relevant information is provided transparently. This principle reinforces the importance of treating individuals with autonomy and respect throughout the research process, safeguarding their dignity at every stage.

5.4.3.1 Right to Self-Determination

Individuals should be recognized as autonomous beings, capable of making their own decisions and controlling their actions. Self-determination allows potential participants to voluntarily choose whether or not to participate in a study, without fear of bias or negative consequences. It also grants them the right to ask questions, decline to provide certain information, and withdraw from the study at any point.

An individual's right to self-determination includes protection from **coercion**, which can arise from threats of penalties for refusing to participate or the promise of excessive incentives for agreeing to take part in a study. Safeguarding participants from coercion is particularly important when the researcher holds a position of authority or influence, as is often the case in nurse-patient relationships. However, the risk of coercion should also be carefully considered in situations where no prior relationship exists. It is crucial to ensure that participants are not influenced by external pressures. For instance, in a clinical setting, offering faster or preferential medical treatment to patients in exchange for their participation could be seen as mildly coercive. Patients might feel compelled to participate, fearing that declining could delay their care or lead to less favorable treatment. In such cases, researchers must ensure that patients' decisions to participate are entirely voluntary and free from concerns about their healthcare.

5.4.3.2 Right to Disclosure

The right to disclosure is a fundamental ethical principle in research, requiring that participants receive all relevant information necessary to make informed, voluntary decisions about their involvement in a study. Full disclosure in research includes informing participants about the study's purpose, procedures, potential risks, and benefits as well as their right to decline or withdraw from participation at any point. This transparency is crucial for building trust and ensuring participants can fully exercise their right to self-determination. Providing a clear explanation of the researcher's responsibilities and the potential consequence of participation ensures that the informed consent process is upheld, protecting participants' **autonomy** and maintaining high ethical standards in research. Honest and open communication throughout the process is key to ensuring ethical and voluntary participation.

Full disclosure can be challenging in nursing studies as it may introduce bias and affect recruitment. For example, if a study aimed to assess whether long nursing shifts lead to more medication errors, fully revealing the purpose might deter nurses who have made errors from participating or lead them to alter their behavior. This could skew the results and compromise the study's integrity. In such cases, researchers must balance transparency with minimizing influence on participants' responses to ensure valid data.

The **Participant Information Sheet (PIS)** is a crucial document that provides potential participants with all the information they need to make informed, voluntary decisions about joining a study. It outlines the study's purpose, procedures, risks, benefits, and participants' right to withdraw at any time. Additionally, the PIS explains how data will be collected, stored, and kept **confidential**, ensuring transparency and protecting participants' privacy.

Including clear information and contact details for the research team, the PIS allows participants to ask questions and seek clarification before consenting to participate. This document ensures that participants fully understand the study, reinforcing the importance of informed consent and voluntary participation.

5.4.4   Justice

The principle of justice emphasizes the importance of **fair** treatment for all participants and the protection of their **privacy**. It ensures that no group is unfairly burdened or excluded, and that the benefits and risks of the research are distributed equitably. Upholding **justice** is crucial for maintaining the ethical integrity of a study, ensuring participants are treated with respect and their rights are protected throughout the research process.

5.4.4.1 Right to Fair Treatment

An important element of justice is the fair distribution of both the benefits and burdens of research. Participants should be selected based on the study's requirements rather than on their vulnerability or social standing. Historically, ethical concerns have arisen when researchers targeted disadvantaged groups, such as the poor or prisoners, for participation. The principle of justice places specific obligations on researchers to protect individuals who may be unable to safeguard their own interests, such as terminally ill patients, ensuring that they are not exploited or unfairly burdened in the research process. Ethical research practices must prioritize the protection and fair treatment of all participants.

Distributive justice mandates that no individuals or groups who may benefit from research are neglected or discriminated against. It also seeks to ensure that the risks and benefits of research are shared equitably among all participants. A breach of this principle occurred during the Bial drug trial in France, where a phase I clinical trial resulted in the death of one volunteer and neurological harm to others [10]. The trial raised significant ethical concerns, particularly regarding how quickly participants were informed of the risks and how promptly authorities were notified. The delay in communication reflected a failure to protect participants and highlighted the need for justice, which demands that participants are treated with fairness, transparency, and respect, particularly when they are in vulnerable positions. This case underscores the importance of

justice in ensuring ethical treatment and protection in all stages of clinical research.

The principle of fair treatment extends beyond the selection of participants. It ensures that researchers treat individuals who choose not to participate or withdraw from a study without prejudice. Researchers are also obligated to uphold all commitments made to participants, including payment of any promised stipends. Additionally, they must show respect for the beliefs, customs, and lifestyles of individuals from diverse backgrounds or cultures. Fair treatment requires that participants have access to research staff for clarification when needed and that they are treated with courtesy and tact throughout the research process. Upholding this principle is crucial for maintaining trust and ethical integrity in research.

5.4.4.2 Right to Privacy

Research involving human participants often requires accessing personal information, and researchers must take care to minimize intrusions into participants' private lives. It is essential that the research only gathers the information necessary for the study and that participants' privacy is protected at all times. Participants have the right to expect that their personal data will be handled with the utmost confidentiality, ensuring their privacy is respected throughout the research process. Maintaining this privacy is fundamental to ethical research practices and helps build trust between participants and researchers.

One of the primary methods for protecting privacy is through **anonymity** or other confidentiality measures. Anonymity ensures that even the researcher cannot link participants to their data. For example, if nursing staff complete questionnaires without personal identifiers, their responses are anonymous. Likewise, if a researcher reviews shift reports with all identifying details removed, anonymity protects their privacy. Another example is assigning coded numbers in focus group discussions to maintain confidentiality.

Researchers should always aim to achieve anonymity whenever possible. In cases where anonymity is not feasible, it is essential to implement proper **confidentiality** procedures. A confidentiality agreement ensures that any information participants provide will not be publicly disclosed in a way that identifies them, nor will it be accessible to unauthorized individuals. This means that research data should not be shared with strangers or individuals known to the participants (e.g., family members, healthcare providers, or colleagues), unless explicit permission has been granted by the participant. Additionally, safeguarding confidentiality requires researchers to establish secure storage and data management practices to prevent unauthorized access.

5.5   Informed Consent

Informed consent is the process by which a fully informed, competent individual voluntarily decides whether to participate in research. It involves explaining the study, the tasks required, how data will be managed, and participants' rights. This ongoing process begins before signing the consent form and continues throughout the study. Participants must fully understand the research procedures, risks, benefits, and their voluntary participation. The informed consent document, along with an information sheet, ensures participants understand their role and offers legal protection to researchers. This process emphasizes ethical transparency and respect for participants' autonomy.

5.5.1   Definition of "Informed Consent"

The concept of informed consent was first formally outlined in the Nuremberg Code, which states: "The individual must possess the legal capacity to consent, be in a position to exercise free and independent choice without any form of force, fraud, deceit, duress, overreaching, or other coercive elements, and have adequate knowledge and understanding of the subject matter to make an informed and thoughtful decision" [1]. The Nuremberg Code's definition of informed consent has laid the foundation for discussions on consent in all subsequent research codes and

is widely accepted within the research community. Informed consent entails the researcher providing essential information while ensuring that the potential participant is mentally capable and able to understand it. Moreover, participation must be completely voluntary.

Informed consent is a fundamental ethical requirement, ensuring that individuals fully comprehend the implications of their participation and are free from any external pressures that could compromise their autonomy in decision-making.

5.5.2   Essential Participant Information

Prior to an individual with an impairment consenting to participate in a research study, the researcher must ensure the participant is fully informed about the following key elements. It is critical that this information is communicated in a clear and accessible manner, ensuring that the participant fully understands their role in the study. Additionally, the researcher should take extra care to address any questions or concerns the participant may have to ensure they are making an informed and voluntary decision. Providing adequate time for reflection and discussion with family or trusted individuals is equally important to uphold ethical standards in the consent process.

1. *Purpose of Research:* The researcher must explicitly outline the purpose or objectives of the research, explaining the reasons behind conducting the study. Additionally, the researcher should provide a detailed overview of the research procedures, particularly highlighting any experimental aspects. This ensures that participants fully understand what the study entails and how it differs from routine treatments or interventions they might otherwise receive.
2. *Research Procedures:* It is essential to describe the tasks and procedures from the participant's perspective, outlining what will be required of them and specifying the **fre-**

quency and **duration** of each procedure. The researcher must provide an estimate of the total **time** participants will need to commit as well as any additional costs or charges related to the procedures. **Eligibility** criteria should also be clearly stated, explaining why the individual is eligible to participate and the standards used to assess their suitability. By providing this comprehensive information, participants can better understand their role and the extent of their involvement in the study, ensuring they make informed choices about participation.

3. *Potential Risks:* The researcher must explain the possible risks or discomforts participants may face, including minor inconveniences, confidentiality concerns, and any serious adverse effects. The likelihood of these risks, particularly for invasive procedures, should be clearly outlined. Additionally, the researcher must ensure that participants understand the risks, considering that individual perceptions may vary. If participants ask about potential risks, the researcher must provide a detailed explanation.

4. *Potential Benefits:* The researcher should describe any realistic benefits to participants or others without overpromising. If no benefits exist, this should be clearly stated. Compensation terms, including conditions for partial or no payment, must be outlined and comply with relevant policies. Additionally, the potential broader benefits to society or the field should be noted.

5. *Alternatives to Participation:* Participants should be informed of any alternative treatments or procedures that may be beneficial, including standard treatments for their condition. In non-therapeutic research, the main alternative may be opting not to participate.

6. *Levels of Confidentiality:* Although complete confidentiality cannot be guaranteed, steps will be taken to protect participants' privacy. The researcher will explain how confidentiality will be maintained, such as using numeric codes for data, and under what circumstances records may be accessed. Participants will be informed of legal require-

ments for disclosure, such as cases of abuse or criminal activity. In small studies or those using recordings, anonymity may be limited. For focus groups, participants should avoid sharing discussions, but the risk of others doing so must be acknowledged.

7. *Disclosure of Potential Conflict of Interest:* The researcher must inform participants of any potential conflicts of interest and explain how they are being managed to prevent bias or undue influence on the research.

8. *Treatment for Research-Related Injury or Stress:* Participants must be given contact details for the research team and support services in case of injury or adverse events and be assured that timely and appropriate treatment will be provided if necessary.

9. *Right to Withdraw:* Prospective participants should be informed that, even after giving consent, they have the right to withdraw from the study or withhold specific information at any time without penalties. Researchers must clearly explain any risks, limitations, or potential implications of withdrawal and emphasize that doing so will not affect the participant's benefits, services, or standing.

10. *Data Handling and Protection:* Researchers must explain how participant data will be used, whether for publications, future studies, or stored in an archive. If quotes or personal information are included, participants must be informed. Data must be securely stored according to regulations, and participants should be told how long it will be kept. The consent form should be clear, and participants should have enough time to understand the research before deciding to participate.

11. *Ensuring Readability:* The consent document must be clear and easy to understand, using simple, straightforward language and avoiding jargon or technical terms. If technical terms are necessary, they should be clearly defined. To ensure readability, the document should be reviewed by someone not involved in the research to identify any confusing sections. If the participant does

not understand the language, a translated version or interpreter must be provided.

12. ***Ensuring Participant Understanding:*** Researchers must ensure participants understand their role by reviewing the consent document and answering questions. Open-ended questions should be used to gauge understanding, encouraging ongoing dialogue. Participants should be reminded they can ask questions anytime, but it's the researcher's responsibility to provide all necessary information for informed decisions.

13. ***Time for Decision-Making:*** Participants should be given sufficient time to reflect on their decision and consult others before agreeing to participate.

14. ***Contact Information:*** Researchers should provide the names and contact details of the principal investigator, and any student researchers involved. The contact information of a neutral third party should also be given to explain participants' rights and address any concerns.

Essential participant information is fundamental to conducting ethical research. Ensuring participants understand their rights, the study's purpose, and the procedures involved is key. Providing clear details, sufficient time for consideration, and accessible contacts for support fosters trust and transparency, safeguarding participant autonomy and well-being throughout the research process.

5.5.3   Vulnerable Research Participants

The Declaration of Helsinki states that vulnerable groups and individuals are "may have an increased likelihood of being wronged or of incurring additional harm" [3]. Vulnerability refers to a significant inability to safeguard one's own interests due to barriers such as an inability to provide informed consent, limited access to essential services like medical care, or holding a lower or subordinate position within a hierarchical structure [11].

Typically, vulnerable individuals or populations are those whose ability to make informed decisions and safeguard their rights is limited due to factors such as their mental, social, economic, or ethnic status, age, or health condition. In other words, they are at a higher risk of harm in research settings because of these vulnerabilities. Although adhering to ethical standards is typically straightforward, special precautions must be taken to protect the rights of vulnerable groups. These groups may be unable to give fully informed consent or may face increased risk of unintended side effects due to their circumstances.

Researchers working with high-risk populations should become well-versed in the guidelines surrounding informed consent, risk/benefit assessments, and appropriate research methods for these groups. In general, research involving vulnerable subjects should only be pursued when the risk/benefit ratio is low or when no alternative exists. Nurse researchers, in particular, should remain especially vigilant when conducting research involving vulnerable populations. A brief discussion of the four main vulnerable groups is as follows:

5.5.3.1 Children

Children are considered a vulnerable group in research due to their developing decision-making abilities. Many countries have laws regulating their involvement, and Research Ethics Committees must be familiar with relevant regulations, especially for externally funded studies. Special care is needed to protect children's rights, including obtaining parental consent and providing age-appropriate information.

5.5.3.2 Individuals with Intellectual or Mental Disabilities

Individuals with mental disabilities may be unable to provide informed consent, requiring consent from a legal guardian or caregiver. However, like in research with children, appropriate information should still be provided, and assent should be obtained when possible. The research must directly address issues relevant to this group and be necessary to conduct with them. Researchers must ensure that the study cannot be completed with participants without mental disabilities and should prioritize respect, dignity, and clear communication throughout the process.

5.5.3.3 Pregnant Women

Pregnant women may face risks in clinical research due to hormonal changes and potential impacts on the unborn baby. Certain activities can increase the risk of miscarriage, so extra precautions are necessary. While the assumption that pregnant women are inherently vulnerable in giving consent has been debated, their autonomy must be respected. Research Ethics Committees require that pregnant women only participate in studies addressing their specific health needs, with minimal risks to both the mother and fetus, ensuring safety remains the top priority.

5.5.3.4 Prisoners

Prisoners are a vulnerable research population due to their limited ability to make voluntary decisions without coercion. Research Ethics Committees reviewing studies involving prisoners must ensure that most members have no connection to the prison system, but at least one member must represent prisoners' interests, such as a former prisoner. The same criteria of relevance and necessity for vulnerable groups apply, with added care to ensure participation is entirely voluntary.

5.5.3.5 Special Groups

Many groups face stigmatization and selecting them for research can risk worsening their marginalization. Extra safeguards must be in place to prevent participants from being identified by their communities. Stigmatizing characteristics may include conditions like albinism, infertility, sexual orientation, or certain cultural practices. Vulnerable groups, such as commercial sex workers and substance abusers, face similar risks. Research Ethics Committees must ensure that researchers respect participants and minimize potential harm. Handling sensitive information—such as racial or ethnic origin, health conditions,

or criminal behavior—requires careful consideration to prevent negative consequences for participants.

5.6 Research Misconduct

Ethical research not only ensures the protection of human and animal subjects but also preserves public trust in the scientific process. In recent years, concerns about research misconduct, including fraud and misrepresentation, have grown. Definitions of research misconduct vary between countries and institutions, often based on the intent and seriousness of the actions. Despite the lack of a universal definition, the U.S. Office of Research Integrity provides one of the most widely accepted descriptions, defining research misconduct as "fabrication, falsification, or plagiarism in proposing, conducting, reviewing, or reporting research results." These actions represent significant breaches of ethical standards and undermine the credibility and integrity of scientific research. Maintaining rigorous ethical oversight is essential to safeguarding the reliability of scientific inquiry.

- **Fabrication** involves creating false data or results and presenting them as legitimate findings in research records or reports.
- **Falsification** refers to altering research materials, equipment, processes, or manipulating data in a way that distorts the research, leading to inaccurate representation in the final report.
- **Plagiarism** is the act of using someone else's ideas, methods, results, or words without proper acknowledgment or attribution.

Although fabrication, falsification, and plagiarism are the officially recognized forms of misconduct, other unethical practices also constitute research misconduct. These include improper authorship, inadequate data management, conflicts of interest, non-compliance with regulations, and unauthorized use of confidential information. Conflicts of interest, especially in health research funded by for-profit organizations, are a particularly pressing issue that must be carefully managed to uphold the integrity of research. Ensuring transparency and accountability in these areas is essential for maintaining trust in scientific findings.

Research misconduct clearly undermines the validity and credibility of scientific research [12, 13]. However, breaches in research integrity are not limited to major offenses; they can also involve less severe actions often referred to as questionable research practices (QRPs).

QRPs often occupy a gray area in research ethics and are not fully understood. In some cases, QRPs cause direct and tangible harm, such as negatively impacting medical care or wasting research funds. In other instances, the harm is more subtle, as QRPs can lead to irreproducible findings, delay the detection of misconduct, hinder the correction of erroneous results, and contribute to inadequate training for students. These issues underscore the significant impact of QRPs on the research process. These minor misbehaviors, while less egregious, still pose significant risks to the integrity of research.

An increasing number of studies highlight violations of scientific norms and a lack of research integrity across various scientific disciplines. A recent systematic review and meta-analysis by [14] found that 2.9% of researchers admitted to committing research misconduct, such as falsification, fabrication, or plagiarism (FFP), while 12.5% reported engaging in at least one instance of QRPs. Additionally, 15.5% of researchers observed colleagues engaging in FFP, and 39.7% were aware of others using QRPs. These findings underscore the widespread nature of research misconduct and the need for more robust ethical oversight, highlighting the under-reporting of misconduct in self-reports and emphasizing the importance of rigorous monitoring and accountability measures in research.

5.7   Institution Review

Institutional Review Boards (IRBs) or research ethics committees are essential for protecting human research participants by conducting independent reviews of the ethical acceptability of research proposals. They are responsible for ensuring that proposed research meets ethical standards, monitoring potential biases of clinical investigators, and verifying compliance with laws and regulations designed to safeguard human subjects. Many countries around the world require such independent reviews. IRBs or ethics committees, made up of individuals not directly involved in the research, review study plans and documents before the study begins and periodically thereafter, usually on an annual basis, throughout the study's duration.

The primary goal of IRB review is to ensure that the rights and welfare of research participants are adequately protected. To meet ethical and regulatory standards, IRBs assess that the risks to participants are minimized and are reasonable in relation to the potential knowledge the study may generate. They also ensure that participant selection is fair, with clear inclusion and exclusion criteria, and that informed consent procedures are appropriately planned. This thorough review process ensures that human subjects are protected throughout the course of the research.

An IRB has the authority to approve, require modifications to, or disapprove proposed research plans. The key criteria guiding IRB decisions can be summarized as follows: risks to participants must be minimized, and the risks involved should be reasonable in relation to any potential benefits and the importance of the knowledge the study is expected to generate. Additionally, the selection of participants must be fair and equitable, ensuring that all individuals are chosen without bias.

Informed consent is another crucial factor; it must be obtained as required and appropriately documented. Adequate provisions must also be in place to monitor the research and ensure participant safety throughout the study. Further, steps must be taken to protect participants' privacy and to ensure the confidentiality of their data. If vulnerable groups are part of the study, additional safeguards are required to protect their rights and welfare. These criteria help ensure that research is carried out ethically, with a strong focus on participant protection and compliance with legal and ethical standards.

IRBs are crucial in safeguarding human research participants from potential harm and exploitation. Through independent oversight, they ensure ethical standards are adhered to and that proper protections are in place to secure the rights and welfare of participants. This oversight is a key component of a larger system designed to promote ethical and scientifically valid research while protecting those involved. Moreover, IRBs play a pivotal role in maintaining public confidence by ensuring transparency and accountability throughout the research process.

References

1. International Military Tribunal. Trials of war criminals before the nuremberg military tribunals under Control Council Law No. 10, Nuernberg, October 1946–April 1949. U.S. Government Printing Office; 1949.
2. World Medical Association. WMA Declaration of Helsinki: ethical principles for medical research involving human subjects. Adopted by the 18th WMA General Assembly, Helsinki, Finland; June 1964.
3. World Medical Association. World Medical Association Declaration of Helsinki: ethical principles for medical research involving human subjects. JAMA. 2013;310(20):2191–4.
4. Henderson V. An overview of nursing research. Nurs Res. 1957;6(2):61.
5. Stievano A, Tschudin V. The ICN code of ethics for nurses: a time for revision. Int Nurs Rev. 2019;66(2):154–6.
6. ICN. The ICN code of ethics for nurses. Revised 2021 [Internet]. Geneva: International Council of Nurses; 2021. p. 1–32. https://www.icn.ch/sites/default/files/2023-06/ICN_Code-of-Ethics_EN_Web.pdf.
7. National Commission for the Protection of Human Subjects of Biomedical and Behavioral, Research. The Belmont report: ethical principles and guidelines for the protection of human subjects of research. Washington, DC: The Commission; 1979.
8. Pitney W, Parker J, Mazerolle S, Potteiger K. Qualitative research in the health professions. New York: Taylor & Francis; 2024.
9. Godskesen T, Björk J, Juth N. Challenges regarding informed consent in recruitment to clinical research: a qualitative study of clinical research nurses' experiences. Trials. 2023;24(1):801.
10. Casassus B. France releases interim report on drug trial disaster. Lancet. 2016;387(10019):634–5.
11. CIOMS. Guideline 15: research involving vulnerable persons and groups. International ethical guidelines for health-related research involving humans. Council for International Organizations of Medical Sciences. 4th ed. Geneva: World Health Organization; 2016. p. 1–199.
12. Bhaskar R, Ola M. Publication misconduct, plagiarism, and research integrity. Principles of research methodology and ethics in pharmaceutical sciences. Boca Raton: CRC Press; 2024.
13. Narang U, Kurian NK. Editorial misconducts: boosting citation and impact factor. In: Joshi PB, Churi PP, Pandey M, editors. Scientific publishing ecosystem: an author-editor-reviewer axis [Internet]. Singapore: Springer Nature; 2024. p. 213–31. https://doi.org/10.1007/978-981-97-4060-4_13.
14. Xie Y, Wang K, Kong Y. Prevalence of research misconduct and questionable research practices: a systematic review and meta-analysis. Sci Eng Ethics. 2021;27(4):41.

Evidence-Based Practice in Nursing

6

Learning Outcomes

By the end of this chapter, readers should be able to:

1. Understand the fundamental principles and evolution of evidence-based practice (EBP) in nursing.
2. Explain the hierarchy of evidence and its significance in guiding clinical decision-making.
3. Identify and describe various EBP models and frameworks used in healthcare, such as the Iowa and Johns Hopkins models.
4. Analyze the challenges associated with implementing EBP in clinical settings and propose strategies to overcome them.
5. Evaluate the impact of EBP on patient outcomes and its role in advancing nursing practice.

6.1   Introduction

Evidence-based practice (EBP) is now broadly acknowledged as a critical component in enhancing healthcare quality and improving patient outcomes. Although the primary goals of nursing research to create new knowledge and evidence-based nursing practice to implement the best available evidence might appear separate, there is increasing acknowledgment of their strong interconnection. Increasingly, research studies are being designed with a focus on translating evidence into practical application in clinical settings. It is evident that for research-driven innovations to be truly impactful, they must be paired with effective implementation strategies and supported by a conducive environment.

EBP has its origins in medicine, thanks to British epidemiologist Archie Cochrane. He criticized the medical profession for failing to critically evaluate treatments and argued that healthcare should be based solely on scientific evidence [1]. Cochrane advocated for randomized clinical trials as the gold standard for reliable evidence and called for systematic reviews from various disciplines to guide practice and policy. His efforts led to the creation of the Cochrane Center, promoting evidence-informed decision-making [2]. Over time, EBP in medicine evolved to include not only research evidence but also clinical judgment and patient preferences.

The term "evidence-based practice" (EBP) emerged from the concept of evidence-based medicine (EBM) and has since been adopted across various professional fields, including nursing. Since the integration of EBP into nursing, there has been a global consensus on the importance of healthcare providers incorporating research evidence into their practice. Evidence-based care is associated with numerous benefits, including enhanced healthcare quality, improved safety, and reduced care costs. However, despite significant progress over the past three decades, challenges remain in fully understanding and consistently implementing EBP in practice. To address these gaps, further efforts are needed to standardize the application of EBP and improve education and training for healthcare providers.

Over the past three decades, significant progress has been made toward integrating this concept into healthcare. However, evidence indicates ongoing challenges in fully understanding EBP and inconsistencies in its implementation across clinical settings. This highlights the need for continued efforts to ensure that evidence-based care is consistently applied in practice.

6.1.1   Definition of EBP

Despite the variety of terminologies associated with EBP, such as discipline-specific terms like evidence-based nursing and evidence-based medicine, the core purpose and key principles remain consistent across fields. Evidence-based medicine is defined as the "conscientious, explicit, and judicious use of current best evidence in making decisions about the care of individual patients." This approach requires integrating clinical expertise with the most reliable external evidence obtained from systematic research [3]. Ultimately, this practice ensures that patient care is informed by both expert judgment and the best available scientific data, fostering more effective and personalized treatment decisions.

Although this definition highlights the importance of integrating the best available evidence with clinical expertise, a key criticism is that it initially overlooked the perspectives of service users, as previously noted by Melnyk and Fineout-Overholt [4]. A more comprehensive definition of EBP now encompasses a three-pronged approach, which includes the best current evidence, clinical expertise, and patient values and preferences. The International Council of Nurses (ICN) emphasizes that "evidence-based practice is a problem-solving approach to clinical decision-making that incorporates a search for the best and latest evidence, clinical

expertise and assessment, and patient preferences and values, within a context of caring" [5].

Similarly, evidence-based nursing is defined as the "conscientious, explicit, and judicious use of theory-derived, research-based information in making decisions about care delivery to individuals or groups of patients, reflective of individual needs and preferences" [6]. This evolving definition reinforces the importance of patient-centered care, ensuring that treatment plans are not only evidence-based but also tailored to the unique needs and preferences of each patient. All these definitions emphasize the conscientious use of the best available evidence to guide decisions about patient care. Over time, the definition of EBP has evolved into a broader, lifelong problem-solving approach to clinical practice, incorporating several essential elements.

These elements include a systematic search for, critical appraisal of, and synthesis of the most relevant and high-quality research to address key clinical questions. It also involves integrating one's own clinical expertise, which includes internal evidence from outcomes management, quality improvement initiatives, thorough patient assessments, and the effective use of available resources to achieve optimal patient outcomes.

Additionally, EBP considers patient preferences and values in the decision-making process. Unlike research utilization, which often focuses on applying findings from a single study, EBP synthesizes evidence from multiple studies, blending research with the clinician's expertise and the patient's unique preferences to provide more comprehensive and individualized care [7, 8]. This expanded definition underscores the importance of continuously enhancing clinical practice by combining evidence with experience and patient-centered care.

The primary reason for adopting an evidence-based approach in practice is to improve the quality of care for patients and achieve better outcomes. This approach not only enhances patient care but also provides a structured framework that supports decision-making and helps healthcare professionals make informed judgments [9]. Through the use of EBP, nurses become more adept at asking relevant questions about changes in their care methods and are better equipped to assess and refine their practices. Additionally, this approach has the potential to lower healthcare costs through the implementation of more efficient, targeted interventions [10, 11]. Furthermore, an evidence-based approach fosters a culture of continuous improvement, ensuring that patient care evolves in line with the latest and most reliable research.

6.2 Hierarchy of Evidence

The hierarchy of evidence is a structured framework used to classify various types of research according to their strength, reliability, and susceptibility to bias [8]. This system plays a crucial role in helping clinicians and researchers identify the most trustworthy evidence to guide decision-making in clinical practice. Since different types of evidence vary in their resistance to errors and biases, it is essential to understand where a study falls within this hierarchy in order to make informed, evidence-based decisions.

This framework prioritizes high-quality research while acknowledging the inherent limitations of lower levels of evidence.

At the top of the hierarchy are umbrella reviews, which synthesize multiple systematic reviews and meta-analyses, offering a comprehensive and reliable overview of a particular topic with minimal bias (Fig. 6.1) [12]. As these reviews integrate findings from numerous high-quality studies, they provide the strongest form of evidence, serving as a key resource for clinical decision-making.

Following umbrella reviews are systematic reviews and meta-analyses. Systematic reviews critically assess and synthesize the findings of multiple studies, while meta-analyses statistically combine the data from these studies to draw reliable and robust conclusions. If based on randomized controlled trials, these methods offer a high level of evidence that is crucial for guiding both clinical research and practice.

The hierarchy, as depicted in Fig. 6.1, ensures that the most reliable and least biased forms of evidence are prioritized in clinical and organiza-

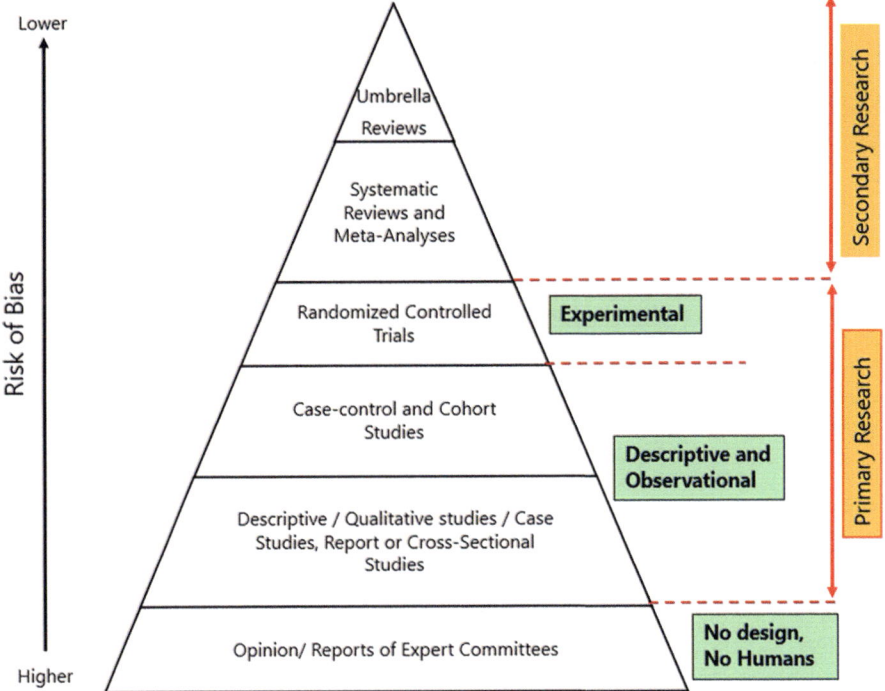

Fig. 6.1 Hierarchy of evidence

tional decisions. Through following this structured approach, clinicians can make more accurate and informed decisions, ultimately improving patient outcomes and advancing the field of evidence-based practice.

6.3   Steps of Evidence-Based Practice

One way to manage the complexity of EBP in healthcare is through the development of specific EBP models and frameworks. These frameworks provide a structured approach for translating evidence into clinical practice, allowing organizations to evaluate their readiness and willingness to implement changes within complex healthcare systems [13]. Supporting organizations in identifying resource needs, barriers, and facilitators, EBP models guide the entire implementation process, ensuring that evidence-based interventions are effectively integrated into practice.

Although numerous scoping reviews have been published on implementation science, there is a lack of a comprehensive review specifically focused on EBP models and frameworks. In a recent scoping review, **19** EBP models and frameworks used in healthcare settings were identified [14]. These models vary significantly in their approach to translating research into practice. For instance, some, such as the Iowa [15] and Johns Hopkins models [16], provide detailed tools and resources for implementation, whereas others, like the ACE Star model [17], offer a more generalized overview.

The inclusion of patient values, preferences, and clinical skills also differs among the models. Frameworks such as the Advancing Research and Clinical practice model [18] and Joanna Briggs Institute Model [19] incorporate patient values into their processes, whereas others only acknowledge this aspect without providing clear guidance on its integration Table 6.1. Additionally, the review highlighted gaps in clinician expertise in appraising evidence, with many models recommending the involvement of EBP mentors to guide this critical step. Only a few models offer comprehensive methods for evaluating the success of implemented changes. Despite the diversity of these models, the level of support and

Table 6.1 Models and framework of EBP steps

Lowa [15]	Johns' Hopkins models [16]	ACE Star model [17]	RACC [18]	Joanna Briggs Institute Model [19]
1. Question development	1. Practice question: EBP question is identified	1. Discovery: Searching for new knowledge	1. Assess the healthcare organization for readiness for change	1. Global Health
2. Searches, appraises, and synthesizes the literature	2. Evidence: The team searches, appraises, rates the strength of evidence	2. Evidence summary: Synthesize the body of research knowledge	2. Identify potential and actual barriers and facilitators	2. Evidence generation
3. If literature is lacking, conduct research	3. Translation: Feasibility, action plan and change implemented and evaluated	3. Translation: Provide clinicians with a practice document	3. Identify EBP champions	3. Evidence synthesis
4.Develop, enact and appraise a pilot solution		4. Integration: Changed through formal and informal channels	4. Implement evidence into practice	4. Evidence (knowledge) transfer
5. If successful, implement across organization		5. Evaluation: EBP outcomes are evaluated	5. Evaluate EBP outcomes	5. Evidence implementation
6. If unsuccessful, restart process				

guidance they provide remains inconsistent, reflecting the need for tailored approaches to meet the varying needs of healthcare organizations.

A conceptual framework or model serves as a blueprint for empirical inquiry, constructed from a set of interconnected concepts that are considered essential to the investigation. These concepts work together to define and shape the course of the inquiry or actions taken. In nursing, frameworks have been instrumental in guiding research, establishing the foundation for clinical practice, and informing educational programs. Similarly, models designed for implementing evidence-based practice (EBP) have been developed to direct the process. Although these models differ in their level of detail, specificity, and methods, they share a core set of common steps or phases. These include:

1. **Formulate**: Define the clinical question or problem to be addressed.
2. **Search**: Gather the best available evidence from relevant sources.
3. **Appraise**: Critically assess the quality and relevance of the evidence.
4. **Apply**: Implement the evidence in clinical practice, considering patient preferences and context.
5. **Evaluate**: Continuously monitor and assess the outcomes of the applied evidence to ensure effectiveness.

The steps outlined in this chapter are grounded in both theoretical and research literature, incorporating evidence-based practice, research utilization, and change management theories. These steps provide a comprehensive framework for nurse practitioners, guiding them from the initial assessment of the need for change to the successful implementation and integration of evidence-based protocols into clinical practice. Employing a systematic approach, which involves formulating clinical questions, searching for relevant evidence, appraising its quality, applying it in practice, and evaluating the results, enhances consistency and elevates the standard of care. Through this process, clinical outcomes are

improved, nursing knowledge is advanced, and best practices in the profession continue to evolve.

Additional details on how to incorporate these EBP steps into clinical settings are provided in the following sections, where each step is thoroughly outlined. These sections offer practical guidance to ensure seamless integration of EBP into daily clinical workflows, ultimately enhancing patient care and outcomes.

6.3.1   Formulate

In everyday nursing practice, clinical questions frequently emerge that require evidence-based answers. Clearly identifying the key elements of these questions is an essential first step in guiding nursing decisions or informing research to enhance patient care and outcomes.

The PICO model (Population, Intervention, Comparison, and Outcomes) serves as a practical framework for nurses to develop well-structured, answerable clinical questions Table 6.2.

A well-structured and focused clinical question is more likely to result in a credible and valuable answer, whereas a poorly formulated question can lead to uncertainty and confusion in clinical practice. In nursing, the population and intervention should be specific, but nurses must avoid being overly restrictive. Narrowly defined populations or interventions may limit the avail-

Table 6.2 The PICO format

Population: Who are the relevant patients or the population group facing the issue?
Example: In patients undergoing surgery
Intervention: What nursing intervention or treatment is being considered?
Example: …does using double gloves during surgery…
Comparison: What is the main comparison or alternative to the intervention?
Example: …compared to using a single pair of gloves…
Outcomes: What are the desired outcomes or results of the intervention for the patient? What outcomes are of most importance to the patient or nurse?
Example: …reduce the incidence of surgical site infections and improve postoperative recovery outcomes?

ability of relevant studies or sufficient data to inform EBP. For the population, this may refer to patients with specific health conditions, those at risk of developing a disease, or patients at particular stages of an illness. It can also include defining the clinical context, such as patients in intensive care or those in long-term care.

Nursing interventions can range from preventive measures and screenings to therapeutic treatments or care plans. It is often important to clarify key aspects of the intervention, such as the method of delivery, frequency, dosage, duration, or different components of a comprehensive care plan. The comparison might involve no intervention, a placebo, or different standards of care, and understanding the most appropriate comparator is essential to drawing meaningful conclusions.

Outcomes should focus on what matters most to the patient or nursing care team. These outcomes may include patient comfort, quality of life, or clinical improvements, rather than surrogate markers like lab values, unless they are clearly connected to patient-centered outcomes. For more complex nursing questions, using a logical framework helps clarify the potential pathways and the relationships between interventions and outcomes, ensuring that nurses are equipped to make EBP.

6.3.1.1 Formulating Effective PICO Questions

A strong research question is defined by several key elements that guide the research process effectively. **Clarity** and **specificity** are essential, as the question should be clear, focused, and precisely outline what it aims to investigate. A well-constructed question leaves no room for ambiguity about its scope and purpose, ensuring that the research stays on track and aligns with its intended objectives. The clearer the question, the easier it becomes to design a study that can effectively address it.

Relevance is equally important when crafting a research question. The question should tackle a significant issue or gap within the field, ensuring that the research contributes meaningfully to existing knowledge. Research that addresses a relevant problem has the potential to influence practice, shape future studies, or inform policy.

Furthermore, the **feasibility** of the question must be considered. It needs to be researchable within the practical constraints of time, resources, and available data or methodologies. If a question is too broad or requires inaccessible data, it risks becoming unmanageable or unsustainable.

In addition to being clear and feasible, a good research question should exhibit **originality**. This means exploring an under-researched area or offering a fresh perspective on an established topic. While complete uniqueness is not always necessary, the question should add something new to the discourse, either by challenging existing assumptions or by extending the boundaries of current knowledge. This originality sets the foundation for innovation and progression in the field.

Another vital characteristic is **measurability**. The question must allow for outcomes or data that can be collected and analyzed, ensuring it can be answered through a structured research approach. Without measurability, the research could lead to vague conclusions that are difficult to interpret or apply in practice. Clear, quantifiable outcomes allow researchers to draw solid, evidence-based conclusions.

The **significance** of the research question lies in the contribution it makes to the field. A well-crafted question not only answers an important query but also advances understanding and provides valuable insights. Moreover, the question should generate interest by capturing the attention and curiosity of the target audience or the broader scientific community. An engaging question encourages discussion, sparks further inquiry, and may inspire subsequent research projects.

Lastly, **ethical considerations** must be embedded within the research question. The question should align with ethical guidelines, ensuring that the study will protect the rights and well-being of participants. A research question that overlooks ethical concerns risks undermining the validity and impact of the study, as well as harming participants.

A strong research question is defined by several key elements that guide the research process effectively. Clarity and specificity are essential, as the question should be clear, focused, and precisely outline what it aims to investigate. A well-constructed question leaves no room for ambiguity about its scope and purpose, ensuring that the research stays on track and aligns with its intended objectives. The clearer the question, the easier it becomes to design a study that can effectively address it.

Previous studies have emphasized that a strong research question should be feasible, interesting, novel, ethical, and relevant [20, 21]. Crafting such a question typically requires an iterative process, with multiple revisions and refinements to ensure it meets these critical standards. Each revision helps sharpen the focus, align the question with practical constraints, and ensure that it addresses a gap in the field while adhering to ethical guidelines. Developing a well-defined research question is an essential step toward conducting meaningful and impactful research.

In the absence of a well-constructed question, nurses are likely to encounter irrelevant, excessive, or inaccurate information during their search. Developing the skill to craft a well-formulated question enhances confidence, leading to more efficient and successful searches. Hays et al. [22] identified formulating a clear, searchable, and answerable question as the most challenging aspect of the EBP process. However, they also highlighted additional benefits, such as improving communication of patient information with colleagues, enhancing the understanding of complex content for nursing students, and fostering professional growth by promoting the practice of asking thoughtful questions, finding the best evidence, and making a positive impact on patient care.

Furthermore, numerous web-based resources are available to assist nurses in learning how to develop effective, answerable questions. Investing time in formulating a well-constructed question is invaluable, as it not only sharpens the focus of a search, reducing time spent, but also improves the quality of the results. Crafting a clear and focused question is the first step, and often the most difficult, in providing evidence-based care to patients, but it is essential for ensuring successful outcomes in nursing practice.

6.3.2 Search

The second step in the evidence-based practice (EBP) process is to search for the most reliable evidence. Systematic literature searching is a critical component of EBP, requiring a comprehensive and structured approach to identify relevant studies. This process promotes transparency, allowing readers to understand how studies were identified and how findings are situated within the broader evidence base. Following this method, healthcare professionals can make clinical decisions based on well-documented, high-quality evidence, ensuring accountability and rigor in practice. Additionally, systematic searches help minimize bias by including all relevant studies in the decision-making process.

The search strategy should include the following key steps:

– **Define eligibility criteria and keywords terms:** Establish clear definitions and criteria for selecting relevant studies.
– **Select the right database:** Choose appropriate databases, such as PubMed or the Cochrane Library.
– **Select studies:** Evaluate and choose studies based on their relevance and quality.

A well-structured search ensures that clinical decisions are grounded in the best available evidence, supporting effective and accountable healthcare practices.

6.3.2.1 Define Eligibility Criteria and Keywords Terms

Main Eligibility Criteria
Eligibility criteria are typically derived from the Population, Intervention, Comparison, Outcome (PICO) framework of the review question, along with the specific types of studies that have investigated these elements. The population, interventions, and comparators outlined in the review question generally form the foundation of the eligibility criteria. However, translating these components into clear, practical criteria is not always straightforward and demands careful con-

sideration to ensure that only the most relevant and appropriate studies are included. A thoughtful approach helps to refine the selection process, ensuring that the evidence gathered is robust and directly applicable to the research question. Additionally, clearly defined eligibility criteria enhance the transparency and reproducibility of the review [23].

The first step is to define the broad **population** and setting of interest. This includes determining whether a specific population group fits within the review's scope, based on factors such as age, sex, race, educational status, or the presence of certain conditions [24]. Identifying relevant subpopulations is essential for tailoring the intervention. If such subpopulations are identified, there are two options: either narrow the review's focus to exclude certain subgroups or maintain a broader scope and address subpopulations in the analysis. Additionally, the setting, whether a community, hospital, nursing home, chronic care facility, or outpatient environment, should be specified, as it may significantly impact the intervention's applicability and outcomes.

Defining the **intervention** may be straightforward, but more complex definitions are often required for multi-component interventions involving diverse populations. This complexity arises when considering how the intervention achieves its intended effect and whether variations could lead to different outcomes. The key challenge for review authors is to identify the most critical factors to address.

Clearly defined intervention groups are essential for two main reasons [25]. First, they directly impact the review's findings, ensuring optimal data use and preventing bias. Second, standardized groups help resolve inconsistencies in labeling across studies, improving clarity and accuracy throughout the review process. For example, as illustrated in Table 6.2, the intervention might involve using double gloves during surgery to reduce the risk of infection. How these interventions are grouped and defined plays a significant role in ensuring consistency and reliability in synthesizing findings across studies.

The next critical step is to define the **comparisons** between the intervention groups. Although more complex analyses, such as network meta-analyses, compare multiple groups simultaneously, standard meta-analyses focus on comparing the effects of two groups at a time. These comparisons form the foundation for the synthesis, assuming data are available.

The three common comparisons are: intervention versus placebo (placebo drug or sham procedure, often in pharmacological studies), intervention versus control (no intervention, wait-list, or usual care), and intervention A versus intervention B (comparing two active interventions differing in time, duration, dosage, or type) [24]. The first two comparisons evaluate the effectiveness of an intervention, while the third compares two interventions.

For example, as given in Table 6.2, an intervention might involve using double gloves during surgery. A comparison under the "intervention A versus intervention B" category could be using double gloves versus a single pair of gloves. This highlights the importance of comparing active interventions to determine the most effective approach for patient care.

Outcome domains are determined during the formulation of the PICO question, with defining and grouping outcomes following a process similar to specifying intervention groups. Studies should not be excluded solely because they lack certain outcome data, as this helps avoid bias from selective reporting [26]. However, in some cases, specific outcomes may be necessary for study inclusion. EBP should include outcomes meaningful to both users and recipients of the evidence, covering areas like disease progression, hospital readmission rates, patient-reported outcomes (e.g., pain, quality of life), treatment side effects, and economic impact. Addressing both adverse and beneficial outcomes ensures a comprehensive assessment of the intervention's effectiveness.

For example, as given in Table 6.2, the outcome could focus on reducing surgical site infections and improving postoperative recovery outcomes. In this case, patient-reported outcomes such as pain levels and quality of life could be measured alongside clinical outcomes like reduced infection rates and faster recovery times. These outcomes help assess both the effectiveness and overall impact of the intervention on patient well-being and healthcare resources.

Other Eligibility Criteria

Certain **study designs** are more appropriate for addressing specific research questions. Researchers should carefully select designs that are likely to yield reliable data aligned with their review objectives. The choice of primary research designs (e.g., observational, experimental, controlled, or uncontrolled) must match the type of PICO question and the data synthesis method, such as the need for controlled studies in certain meta-analyses. Study design can also affect the validity of the evidence, with some being more susceptible to bias [27]. A thorough bias assessment is conducted during the critical appraisal phase, regardless of any pre-defined quality criteria. Choosing the right designs ensures that the review's conclusions are based on robust evidence.

One key eligibility criterion in reviews is the **publication status** of studies. An inclusive approach, considering both published and unpublished studies as well as gray literature (e.g., conference papers, reports, theses), helps reduce bias. While published studies are more accessible, they are prone to publication bias, as positive results are more likely to be published. Including unpublished studies and gray literature helps balance this and broaden the evidence base [28]. Excluding these studies without strong justification can narrow the review's scope. Although obtaining unpublished studies can be challenging, the bias introduced by their inclusion is often less concerning than the bias from excluding them. Adopting a strategy that includes all publication types ensures a more comprehensive and accurate review.

Although searching for and analyzing studies in multiple **languages** can be resource-intensive, review authors should consider the potential bias of restricting studies to one language, typically English [27]. Limiting studies by language may exclude valuable research, affecting the review's accuracy and comprehensiveness. Additionally, including studies from various languages helps ensure a more balanced evidence base.

In addition to publication status and language, other eligibility criteria must be considered when conducting a review. Factors such as **sample size, geographical location**, and **timeframe** can also impact the inclusion or exclusion of studies. These criteria ensure that the selected studies are relevant to the research question and provide reliable data. Establishing clear eligibility guidelines helps avoid bias, ensures consistency, and improves the overall quality and validity of the review's findings, as given in Table 6.3 for an example of eligibility criteria.

Table 6.3 Example for eligibility criteria (inclusion and exclusion) based on Table 6.2

Inclusion criteria	Exclusion criteria
Patients undergoing surgery (e.g., general, orthopedic, neurological, cardiac)	Patients not undergoing surgery, or those undergoing minor non-invasive procedures
Use of double gloves during surgery	Unrelated interventions
Comparison between double gloves and single pair of gloves	Comparisons not involving glove use (e.g., different types of antiseptics)
Reduction in surgical site infections and improved postoperative recovery	Outcomes unrelated to infection rates or recovery (e.g., patient satisfaction)
Randomized controlled trials, cohort studies, and observational studies	Case studies, expert opinion articles, or studies with high risk of bias
Published peer-reviewed articles only	Unpublished studies, gray literature, or non-peer-reviewed articles
Studies published in English	Studies published in other than English
Study sample size of more than 50 participants	Studies with fewer than 50 participants
Studies conducted in developed countries	Studies conducted in developing countries or geographically limited regions
Studies published within the last 10 years	Studies published more than 10 years ago

Keywords

Keyword searches are a fundamental approach to identifying relevant literature in research. The effectiveness of a keyword search relies heavily on selecting the right terms to ensure comprehensive and accurate results. Choosing appropriate keywords means selecting words or phrases that reflect the core concepts of your research question. These terms should be broad enough to capture a wide range of relevant studies but specific enough to avoid irrelevant results.

To begin, identify the key concepts from your research question or topic and convert them into search terms. Avoid using action words such as "evaluate" or "assess," as these are typically not used in searches. Instead, focus on nouns or concepts that are central to your study, such as population, intervention, or outcome. Additionally, include synonyms and alternative terms to broaden the scope of your search.

For example, Fig. 6.2 illustrates the various terms related to a study aiming to evaluate whether using double gloves during surgery, compared to a single pair of gloves, reduces the incidence of surgical site infections (SSI) and improves postoperative recovery outcomes. Figure 6.2 maps a range of relevant keywords and synonyms across three main categories:

- Glove types (e.g., double gloving, single glove, glove perforation),
- Surgical procedures (e.g., surgery, operation, surgical treatment),
- Infection and outcomes (e.g., surgical site infection, postoperative outcomes, infection control).

This structured keyword approach ensures comprehensive literature coverage by capturing various terms and synonyms used across studies.

6.3.2.2 Select the Right Database

Selecting the right database is essential for effective research, as it ensures access to reliable,

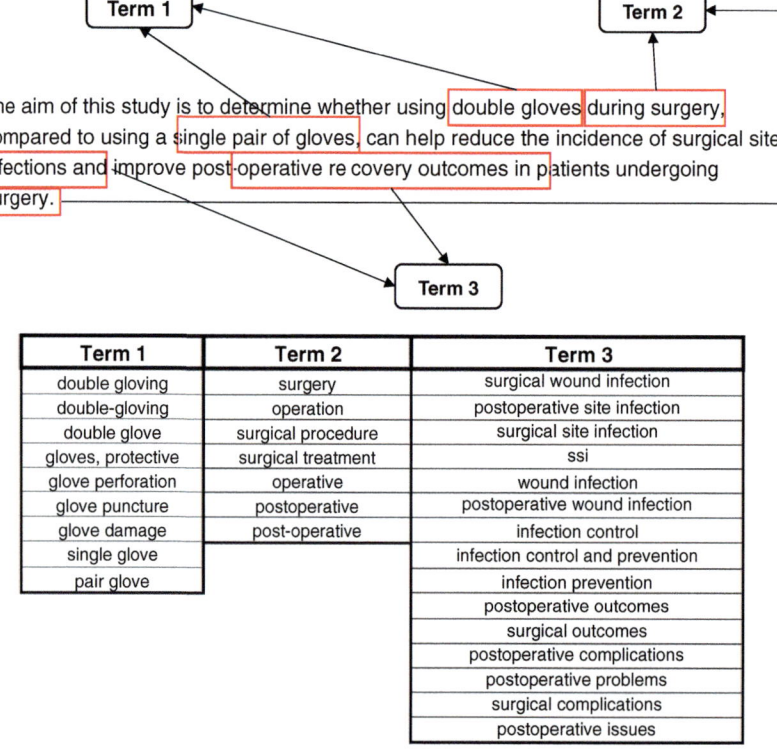

Fig. 6.2 Example for keyword mapping for identifying literature

peer-reviewed, and relevant resources. Start by determining whether your research is general or specialized, and select a database accordingly. Databases differ from search engines like Google and Bing, which provide broad results from the internet. Databases, on the other hand, focus on specific academic fields and offer peer-reviewed, curated content, making them indispensable for accessing structured, high-quality information for specialized research. Selecting the most relevant databases and using multiple sources, you can ensure a comprehensive and reliable literature review. Most higher education institutions and research centers have access to these academic databases, offering a wide range of resources for students and researchers.

Database

Most healthcare professionals rely on the following databases for searching articles:

- PubMed
- Cochrane Databases
- MEDLINE
- CINAHL
- Excerpta Medica Online (EMBASE)
- PsycINFO

These databases provide access to a wide range of peer-reviewed research, clinical studies, and systematic reviews, making them essential resources for evidence-based practice and academic research in healthcare.

PubMed

PubMed is widely regarded as one of the leading bibliographic databases for accessing North American biomedical literature. It hosts and indexes over 27 million citations and articles from MEDLINE and other life science journals, with content dating back to the 1950s. PubMed utilizes Medical Subject Headings (MeSH), a controlled vocabulary system that organizes information under specific subject headings, similar to a dictionary or thesaurus. These headings are structured both alphabetically and hierarchically. While many users begin their searches with basic keywords, this approach may not pro-vide the most thorough results. For more precise and comprehensive searches, it is recommended to consult the MeSH guide to identify the terms that best match or define the search concept. Incorporating these specific subject headings can significantly improve search accuracy and coverage. The link provided, https://pubmed. ncbi.nlm.nih.gov/, is the official website of PubMed.

Cochrane Databases

The Cochrane Collaboration, an international non-profit organization, is supported by a global network of volunteer researchers, healthcare professionals, and consumers. Their efforts focus on preparing, maintaining, and promoting access to six key databases within The Cochrane Library: the Cochrane Database of Systematic Reviews (CDSR), Database of Reviews of Effectiveness (DARE), Cochrane Central Register of Controlled Trials (CENTRAL), Cochrane Methodology Register, Health Technology Assessment Database, and NHS Economic Evaluation Database. Among these, the CDSR is considered the "gold standard" and contains full-text systematic reviews. It is recommended to search this database first when addressing intervention-related questions, as it provides high-quality evidence for healthcare decision-making. The Cochrane Collaboration are accessible through their official website at www.cochrane.org.

MEDLINE

MEDLINE is one of the world's most extensive bibliographic databases, encompassing medicine, health, and the biomedical sciences. Although various platforms, including PubMed, offer different user interfaces, the core content of MEDLINE remains consistent across them. The database indexes citations from over 5200 journals in disciplines such as medicine, nursing, pharmacy, dentistry, and allied health. Updated daily, MEDLINE provides abstracts for more than half of its entries, with 80% of its citations available in English. The link https://www.nlm. nih.gov/medline/medline_home.html is the official website of MEDLINE, maintained by the U.S. National Library of Medicine (NLM).

CINAHL

The Cumulative Index of Nursing & Allied Health Literature (CINAHL) is a comprehensive database produced by Cinahl Information Systems, covering 13 nursing and allied health disciplines. It provides citations, often with abstracts, from a variety of sources such as journals, books, dissertations, drug monographs, and images that may be difficult to find elsewhere. The database contains over three million journal articles from 1982 onward, with around 70% of its citations also available in the MEDLINE database. Like MEDLINE, CINAHL utilizes a controlled vocabulary to improve search accuracy.

CINAHL is particularly popular among nurses, as it indexes over 5000 journals, with more than 770 available in full-text, and holds over 5.5 million records dating back to 1937. Offering a vast collection of nursing and allied health publications, it can be accessed through the EBSCOhost interface and is primarily available through libraries https://www.ebsco.com/de-de/produkte/datenbanken/cinahl-complete.

EMBASE

Excerpta Medica Online (EMBASE) is a major European biomedical and pharmaceutical database, focusing on areas such as drug research, pharmacology, toxicology, clinical medicine, public health, and biomedical engineering. It uses the EMTREE controlled vocabulary and MeSH for indexing. EMBASE contains over 30 million indexed records from more than 6100 peer-reviewed journals, with over two million new articles added annually. Approximately, 80% of the records include full abstracts. Access to EMBASE requires a subscription. The official website can be accessed at https://ospguides.ovid.com/OSPguides/embase.htm.

PsycINFO

PsycINFO is a bibliographic database covering psychology, behavioral sciences, and mental health, with content dating from the late 1800s to the present. It contains over two million citations, including books and dissertations. The database is a key resource for professionals in psychology,

psychiatry, neuroscience, education, nursing, and related healthcare fields https://www.ebsco.com/products/research-databases/apa-psycinfo.

Efficient Search Strategies for Database

During the development of a search strategy, it is essential to keep in mind that most database platforms retrieve results based on the exact terms entered, including any typos. This emphasizes the importance of accuracy and careful selection of search terms. To ensure a comprehensive search, incorporating a variety of relevant keywords and synonyms is necessary. Overlooking alternative terms for a concept may lead to missing key articles, as different authors often use varying terminology for the same idea. Expanding search terms helps capture a broader range of relevant research.

In addition to using selected keywords (in full or truncated form), incorporating index terms into the search is crucial. Index terms, part of a controlled vocabulary in bibliographic databases, categorize papers in a consistent and structured manner, enabling the identification of relevant articles even when different terminology is used. One of the most recognized sets of index terms is Medical Subject Headings (MeSH), used by the National Library of Medicine (NLM) to describe the content of articles indexed in MEDLINE. Combining text words with index terms enhances both the accuracy and scope of search results. One of the most effective strategies is combining keywords using Boolean operators, which many databases support to refine search results. The most commonly used Boolean operators are:

- **OR**—Retrieves results containing either of the search terms, helping to expand the scope of the search. Both free-text keywords and controlled vocabulary terms associated with a concept should be combined using OR to capture all relevant articles, regardless of which term is used.
- **AND**—Finds results that include both search terms, narrowing the search to return only articles containing all specified concepts. Once all necessary information for each con-

cept is located, the terms are combined using AND to focus on studies where all those concepts overlap.

- **NOT**—Filters out unwanted terms, helping to refine the search by excluding specific concepts. This ensures that articles containing the excluded term are removed from the results, allowing for a more focused search.

These operators allow for more precise search results, helping to narrow or broaden the scope of your query as needed.

Additionally, consider using truncation, which involves adding special symbols to a word or its root to increase the chances of finding relevant studies. Typically, Truncation or wildcard operators can be applied to a single term to truncate or identify spelling variations:

- **Asterisk (*)**—retrieves various word endings (e.g., "nurs*" retrieves nurse, nurses, nursing).

- **Question mark (?)**—replaces a single character to capture alternate spellings (e.g., "randomi?ed" retrieves randomized and randomised).

These operators allow for more flexible and comprehensive search results.

For this example, in Table 6.4, the research will report the search terms used as follows:

double gloving OR double gloving OR double glove OR gloves protective OR glove perforation OR glove puncture OR glove damage OR single glove OR pair glove OR glov* **AND** surgery OR operation OR surgical procedure OR surgical treatment OR operative OR postoperative OR postoperative **AND** surgical wound infection OR postoperative site infection OR surgical site infection OR SSI OR wound infection OR postoperative wound infection OR infection control OR infection prevention OR postoperative outcomes OR surgical outcomes OR postoperative complications OR postopera-

Table 6.4 Example of a map of terms for search strategy

Term 1	AND	Term 2	AND	Term 3
Double gloving		Surgery		Surgical wound infection
OR		OR		OR
Double gloving		Operation		Postoperative site infection
OR		OR		OR
Double glove		Surgical procedure		Surgical site infection
OR		OR		OR
Gloves, protective		Surgical treatment		SSI
OR		OR		OR
Glove perforation		Operative		wound infection
OR		OR		OR
Glove puncture		postoperative		Postoperative wound infection
OR		OR		OR
Glove damage		Postoperative		Infection control
OR				OR
Single glove				Infection prevention
OR				OR
Pair glove				Postoperative outcomes
				OR
				Surgical outcomes
				OR
				Postoperative complications
				OR
				Postoperative problems
				OR
				Surgical complications
				OR
				Postoperative issues

tive problems OR surgical complications OR postoperative issues.

These terms and their variations were combined using Boolean operators to ensure a comprehensive search across all relevant topics. After conducting the final search, you can further refine the results by applying filters based on criteria such as publication date, study population, language, full text or other relevant factors suited to the review topic. Most databases offer a range of filters to help narrow down search results according to the specific needs of your research.

After creating a personal account on the database, all research can be saved, allowing for easy access later. Additionally, the saved searches can be rerun at any time using the same keywords, making it convenient to update the results as new items are added to the database. This feature helps ensure that the most current and relevant information is always available. The structure of a search strategy remains consistent, regardless of the platform used to search a database. However, since each major database employs its own controlled vocabulary to index articles, the indexing terms must be adjusted for each database, though key terms typically stay the same across different platforms. These variations in indexing terms are a key reason why it is not recommended to use federated search engines or platforms that search multiple databases simultaneously when conducting a systematic review. Using such platforms can compromise the precision of the search due to differences in how databases index their content.

6.3.2.3 Select Studies

The process of study selection begins after completing both database and manual searches. In this phase, the identified articles are reviewed using predefined inclusion and exclusion criteria to determine their relevance to the research question. This step is critical, as it directly impacts the quality and applicability of the final evidence included in the review.

Once the search results are obtained and exported, typically into an electronic library like EndNote, titles, abstracts, and sometimes full-text articles are carefully screened. At least two reviewers are recommended to assess the studies, ensuring transparency and reproducibility. Using a two-reviewer or group-based approach enhances the reliability of the selection process.

Reviewers often take a cautious approach to ensure no relevant studies are overlooked. If the relevance of a study is unclear from the title or abstract, the full text is obtained for further evaluation. However, this approach can be resource-intensive, as obtaining physical copies or requesting articles from other libraries may be time-consuming and costly. Reviewers must balance thoroughness with efficiency by considering potential delays and costs.

To guide this initial screening phase, the following points are helpful:

- Confirm that the article is published within the time frame specified in the review protocol.
- Ensure that the article is published in a language that meets the inclusion criteria.
- Verify that the study population aligns with the inclusion criteria (e.g., adults, children, or both).
- Assess whether the study addresses the phenomena outlined in the review question.
- Check if the study design is reported and whether it is relevant to the review question.
- Determine if the study measures an outcome relevant to the review.

If the review protocol specifies a particular date range for included papers, studies published outside that range should be excluded unless they are considered primary or seminal sources. In such cases, the review protocol can include a statement allowing the inclusion of these key papers. Once studies are selected for critical appraisal, full-text articles should be thoroughly reviewed, and any that no longer meet the inclusion criteria should be discarded upon further consideration.

This process is essential for narrowing down the most applicable research to answer the review question and ensuring the final selection of studies is both relevant and of high quality.

Transparent Reporting of Search Strategies

The crucial step in conducting a review is to provide a detailed report of the search strategy. This involves outlining any filters applied, such as language or date restrictions, as well as listing the databases and sources consulted. One of the defining aspects of a review is its reproducibility, allowing other researchers to replicate the search process and reach comparable conclusions. Transparent reporting of the search strategy is vital, as it enables readers to evaluate the quality of the search and its sources, ultimately determining the credibility of the review.

To ensure transparency, many journals that publish systematic reviews now follow the PRISMA guidelines (Preferred Reporting Items for Systematic Reviews and Meta-Analyses)—https://www.prisma-statement.org/. These guidelines recommend that the full search strategy for at least one major database be reported in an appendix and published alongside the review. It is insufficient to only list search filters; the methods section must detail all the bibliographic databases searched, including the platform used, the dates of the search, and any limits applied. Additionally, the search results should be clearly reported, often using a flow diagram, as suggested by the PRISMA guidelines, to enhance clarity.

The PRISMA Statement and its extensions are evidence-based recommendations designed to encourage transparent and comprehensive reporting of systematic reviews, scoping reviews, and review protocols. These guidelines serve as a roadmap to help authors clearly describe what was done, what was found, and, in the case of review protocols, what is planned. Following the PRISMA checklist allows authors to provide detailed and structured reporting, which not only informs readers and reviewers about the study's methodology and findings but also enhances the quality of the reporting process. This, in turn, makes the peer review process more efficient and ensures that the study is replicable, a fundamental element of trustworthy research.

6.3.3 Appraise

Critical appraisal is a structured process used to evaluate the quality, credibility, and relevance of research studies, particularly in relation to clinical practice. It requires proficiency in analyzing the strength, significance, and applicability of the evidence, along with an understanding of the context in which the evidence is applied. Merely being published in a peer-reviewed journal does not guarantee the validity of a study's findings; a thorough evaluation of key elements such as study design, research methodology, and data analysis is essential to ensure its reliability.

Critical appraisal involves assessing both the strengths and limitations of research, determining its practical value for guiding clinical decision-making and improving outcomes. Clinicians must balance the strengths and weaknesses of the research rather than focusing solely on flaws, much like how an art appraiser considers multiple factors when evaluating the worth of a painting. This comprehensive evaluation helps determine the study's contribution to evidence-based practice.

Furthermore, critiquing a study is distinct from mere criticism. A critique is an objective and systematic examination of the research, not a personal assessment of the researcher's abilities. This process, often referred to as an "intellectual critique," focuses on the creation itself rather than the creator [29]. The reviewer must remain impartial, avoiding personal opinions and supporting the analysis with relevant research literature. Importantly, since research operates within probabilities and seldom offers absolute certainty, the critique should address the study's apparent strengths, limitations, and findings with careful consideration of its broader implications for practice. Maintaining objectivity, such as avoiding personal pronouns, ensures that the critique is seen as an unbiased evaluation of the research's worth and relevance to clinical practice.

6.3.3.1 Appraisal Tools

Critical appraisal tools and reporting guidelines are indispensable resources for researchers, practitioners, and policymakers engaged in the processes of research and evidence-based practice. Both serve distinct yet interrelated functions, playing crucial roles in guiding evidence-based decision-making and ensuring the integrity of evidence utilized in clinical practice and policy formulation. Employing a systematic approach is essential for assessing key dimensions such as the quality, reliability, validity, methodological rigor, and transparency of the evidence [23]. These factors are pivotal in determining the credibility of research findings and their applicability to practice.

Conducted appropriately, critical appraisal serves to mitigate information overload by enabling researchers to systematically identify credible, unbiased, and relevant evidence. This process ultimately enhances clinical decision-making and informs policy development, ensuring that healthcare interventions and policies are grounded in the most robust evidence available. Critical appraisal, therefore, is not merely a procedural task but a foundational element that supports the integrity of research-based recommendations.

The availability of a diverse array of critical appraisal tools reflects the nuanced demands of different research designs and methodologies. Given the absence of a universally recognized "gold standard" tool, it is imperative that researchers and practitioners select appraisal tools that are tailored to the specific type of evidence under review. While some tools are more generic in scope, others are designed to evaluate specific study designs, such as randomized controlled trials, cohort studies, or qualitative research.

In making this selection, it is essential to review the accompanying documentation and guidelines to ensure the proper use of each tool. Understanding the unique strengths and limitations of each instrument is crucial to the appraisal process. Furthermore, the selection of an appropriate tool requires a thorough understanding of the context in which the study was conducted, the rigor of the research processes employed, and the verifiability of the evidence generated. A well-informed choice of critical appraisal tools ensures

that the findings are not only trustworthy but also applicable to real-world clinical settings and policy frameworks.

6.3.3.2 Critical Appraisal Skills Program (CASP)

The CASP checklists are designed to evaluate various types of studies, providing a structured approach to appraising the quality and rigor of research evidence. The studies that can be assessed using these guidelines include randomized controlled trials, cohort studies, case-control studies, qualitative studies, and systematic reviews [30]. Each checklist is specifically tailored to its respective study design, with questions aimed at assessing the study's validity, methodology, and relevance, ensuring that healthcare professionals can make informed decisions based on robust evidence.

The number of items in each checklist generally ranges from 10 to 12 questions, focusing on essential aspects such as study design, bias, data analysis, and applicability of the results in clinical practice. This methodical evaluation helps guide users in systematically reviewing research quality to enhance their ability to apply evidence-based findings in healthcare settings. For more information, visit the official CASP website at https://casp-uk.net/.

Joanna Briggs Institute (JBI) Critical Appraisal Tools

The JBI provides a robust set of tools designed to appraise the quality of various types of studies, including randomized controlled trials (RCTs), qualitative research, systematic reviews, and economic evaluations. These tools are specifically developed to evaluate the methodological quality of research and determine its relevance and applicability to clinical practice.

Each JBI appraisal tool is tailored to its respective study type, with checklists that include a series of items focusing on essential aspects such as study design, data integrity, validity, bias, and relevance. The number of items in these checklists can vary, typically ranging from 10 to 13 questions depending on the study type, to guide users through a detailed assessment process.

These tools help healthcare professionals systematically evaluate the rigor and credibility of research evidence, ensuring that clinical decisions are well-informed and based on high-quality data. For more details, visit the official JBI website at https://jbi.global/.

Cochrane Risk of Bias Tool

The RoB 2 (Revised Cochrane Risk of Bias Tool) is specifically designed to assess the risk of bias in randomized controlled trials (RCTs). It offers a systematic approach to evaluate various types of bias that can impact the internal validity of RCTs, including selection bias, performance bias, detection bias, attrition bias, and reporting bias. This tool is widely used in evidence-based research to ensure that the findings from RCTs are reliable and free from potential distortions.

The RoB 2 tool comprises a series of structured items that guide the assessment of these biases, typically including around five domains of bias evaluation. Each domain contains specific questions that help reviewers determine the risk level of bias within the trial. The structured nature of this tool supports a transparent and consistent assessment of RCTs, enhancing the credibility of evidence used in clinical guidelines and decision-making. For more details, visit the official resource page at https://methods.cochrane.org/bias/resources/rob-2-revised-cochrane-risk-bias-tool-randomized-trials.

CONSORT (Consolidated Standards of Reporting Trials)

The CONSORT guidelines are specifically designed to improve the reporting of RCTs. These guidelines provide a structured framework to ensure that all aspects of RCTs are transparently reported, including details about study design, participant allocation, intervention delivery, outcome measurement, and data analysis. CONSORT aims to enhance the quality of trial reports, making it easier for readers to assess the validity, reliability, and applicability of the trial's findings.

The CONSORT statement includes a checklist with 25 items that address critical components of RCT reporting. These items guide researchers in clearly describing the methodology, results, and interpretation of their trials, ultimately helping to minimize bias and improve the reliability of published evidence. By adhering to these standards, trial reports become more consistent and comprehensive, supporting evidence-based decision-making in clinical practice. For more details, visit the official CONSORT website https://www.consort-spirit.org/.

GRADE (Grading of Recommendations, Assessment, Development, and Evaluations)

The GRADE system is designed to assess the quality of evidence and the strength of recommendations in healthcare studies. It is primarily used to evaluate evidence from systematic reviews, RCTs, observational studies, and clinical practice guidelines. GRADE is widely applied in developing clinical guidelines, where it helps to formulate recommendations based on the certainty of evidence and the balance between benefits and harms of a particular intervention.

The GRADE system uses a structured approach to rate the quality of evidence across four levels: high, moderate, low, and very low. Although GRADE does not specify a fixed number of items, it considers several critical factors to assess the evidence, including risk of bias, inconsistency of results, indirectness of evidence, imprecision of estimates, and publication bias. These criteria are used to downgrade or upgrade the quality of evidence, guiding the development of recommendations that are either strong or weak based on the overall confidence in the findings. The GRADE approach ensures a transparent and systematic evaluation of the evidence, making it a valuable tool for evidence-based decision-making in clinical practice. The official website can be accessed at https://www.grade-workinggroup.org/.

STROBE (Strengthening the Reporting of Observational Studies in Epidemiology)

The STROBE guidelines are designed to enhance the reporting quality of observational studies, including cohort studies, case-control studies, and cross-sectional studies. STROBE provides a structured checklist that ensures these studies are transparently and thoroughly conducted, making it easier for researchers and healthcare professionals to assess the validity and reliability of the findings.

The STROBE checklist consists of 22 items that cover key elements of study design, data collection, analysis, and interpretation. These items guide researchers in clearly reporting their study's methodology and results, allowing for a more accurate evaluation of the study's strengths and limitations. Adhering to these guidelines, observational studies can present their findings in a consistent and comprehensive manner, facilitating better understanding and utilization of the research evidence. For more details, visit the official STROBE website at https://www.equator-network.org/reporting-guidelines/strobe/.

There are no rigid guidelines for initiating a critical appraisal, but a commonly accepted approach begins by identifying the type of evidence under review—whether primary studies, such as randomized controlled trials, or secondary sources, such as systematic reviews. Once the evidence type is determined, an appropriate appraisal tool is selected. Reviewers then examine the relevant documentation and complete checklists specific to the evidence type to ensure a comprehensive evaluation.

Critical appraisal tools use various metrics to assess the quality of research, focusing on key aspects such as study design and risk of bias. These tools may employ different methods, including ranking and comparing summary scores, evaluating specific components of the manuscript, and qualitatively assessing the research processes that produced the results. Each approach has distinct strengths and contributes to a thorough assessment of research quality. The choice of method should be guided by the study's context and the appraisal's objectives, ensuring that the findings are relevant and applicable to practice.

6.3.3.3 Elements for Evaluation

Critiques are an integral component of EBP and take on various forms, but all critiques share essential elements. The primary purpose of conducting a critique is to assess whether the conclusions of a study are relevant and applicable within the specific context of the clinical setting. This process ensures that the research findings are both useful and appropriate for guiding clinical or organizational decisions. Several key components form the foundation of any critique, providing a structured guide for evaluating the quality, relevance, and utility of research. These elements ensure that evidence is critically appraised, supporting its potential contribution to practice and policy.

For further details on the foundational principles and methodologies critical to conducting thorough critiques, please refer to Chaps. 2 and 3, which offer comprehensive insights into evaluating both quantitative and qualitative research.

6.3.3.4 Aim

The aim of a research study is central to its design, providing the foundation upon which the entire research process is built. A well-defined and clearly articulated aim is essential for guiding the development of research questions, hypotheses, and methodologies. The first step in critiquing a study typically involves identifying and assessing its aim. Key considerations include whether the aim is clear, relevant to practice, and whether the study addresses a clearly articulated need.

In quantitative research, the aim often underpins hypotheses that are tested statistically, particularly in studies involving interventions such as treatments or diagnostic tests. A well-constructed aim specifies the study factors, which are the independent variables controlled by the researcher, as well as the outcome factors, or dependent variables, used to measure results. The clarity of these factors, along with a defined method for measurement, is critical to the study's design. Additionally, the reference population for which the findings are relevant should be clearly stated, ensuring that the study's applicability is understood.

In qualitative research, the aim differs by focusing on "how" and "why" a phenomenon occurs, rather than "what" or "how many." The aim in this context seeks to develop a conceptual or theoretical understanding of the phenomenon in question, often through methods like grounded theory, which is commonly used in health-related research. The aim of qualitative studies guides the investigation into participants' knowledge, experiences, values, attitudes, and emotions, offering deep insights into subjective human experiences.

Study Design

A critical aspect of evaluating research is examining the study's design, as it ensures the research is methodologically sound and aligned with its aims. Designing a robust study requires careful planning to generate evidence that is practical and applicable. A well-considered design, much like a clear set of instructions, helps produce relevant and usable findings, enhancing the credibility and validity of the research. Justifying design choices is essential for ensuring the study's reliability and its potential application in practice.

Study design is crucial in both quantitative and qualitative research, though they are evaluated differently. In quantitative research, designs are ranked based on the "hierarchy of evidence," with randomized controlled trials providing the highest level of reliability and generalizability. In qualitative research, the strength of the evidence is tied to the rigor of data collection and analysis, with techniques like detailed participant selection and data handling playing a key role. While qualitative studies lack a hierarchical ranking system, their credibility depends on the rigorous application of methodology.

Regardless of the research type, the design must address the study's aim, clearly define outcome factors, and target the critical variables. If key outcomes are excluded, the rationale must be clear. A well-constructed design, whether quantitative or qualitative, is essential for generating high-quality evidence that informs practice, supports decision-making, and advances knowledge.

Sampling and Sample Size

Sampling is critical to the validity of any research study, as a sample (n) must represent the larger population (N). In quantitative research, random sampling is often considered the gold standard, as it minimizes bias and enhances the generaliz-

ability of findings (SEEN sampling for Chap. 2). In qualitative research, purposive sampling is most commonly used to gather rich, in-depth data from participants with relevant experiences or knowledge (see Chap. 3).

The required sample size in quantitative studies is typically determined using a formula that accounts for the degree of error tolerated when testing the "null hypothesis," which posits no significant difference between intervention and control groups. Researchers must specify statistical significance (α) and statistical power to ensure the reliability of their results, with 0.05 and 0.8 being common benchmarks. These values should be clearly reported in well-designed studies.

In qualitative research, sample sizes are smaller, often employing purposive sampling to select participants based on specific knowledge or experience. The goal is to achieve depth of understanding rather than breadth. Theoretical sampling may also be used to include multiple perspectives until data saturation is reached, meaning no new information is obtained. Qualitative researchers must justify their participant selection and provide demographic details to enhance the study's credibility. Unlike quantitative studies, where sample size is calculated, qualitative research relies on reaching data saturation to ensure a comprehensive exploration of the topic, leading to credible and insightful findings.

This section will be linked to Chaps. 2 and 3 Direct section and table.

Data Collection

Data collection is a critical component of any research study, as it directly impacts the quality, credibility, and validity of the findings. In quantitative research, data collection methods may include interviews, questionnaires, attitude scales, and observational tools, with questionnaires being the most commonly employed instrument. These are typically structured with closed-ended questions and can be administered through various channels, such as postal surveys, face-to-face interviews, or telephone interviews, each offering specific advantages. Selecting the most appropriate method depends on the study's objectives, and a well-justified choice enhances the rigor and trustworthiness of the research.

Using existing instruments requires researchers to ensure the tool is suitable for measuring the intended concepts. This includes demonstrating the instrument's validity, which refers to its ability to measure what it is intended to, and its reliability, or consistency in measurement. If an instrument is adapted for a new context or population, previously established validity and reliability may not apply, necessitating an explanation of how these factors were reassessed. A pilot study is often recommended to test the instrument's clarity and make necessary adjustments before the full-scale study begins.

A detailed and transparent account of the data collection process is essential for the integrity of any study. This includes specifying the tools used the procedures for data gathering and the methods of analysis. In qualitative research, where data are often collected through interviews, focus groups, or observations, it is important to address potential biases and ensure that the data collection process upholds the credibility of the findings. Furthermore, ethical considerations must be rigorously adhered to, ensuring the protection of participants and the integrity of the research process.

Data Analyses

Evaluating the statistical methods used in data analysis is a crucial aspect of assessing the validity and reliability of research findings. In quantitative research, it is essential that the chosen statistical tests are appropriate for the research question and that the results are accurately presented. The correct application of parametric or nonparametric tests enhances the precision of the findings, while careful attention to potential biases and confounding variables ensures the credibility of the results. Transparent reporting of these methods allows for replication and ensures the rigor of the study. When necessary, consultation with a statistician can provide further assurance regarding the appropriateness of the analytical approach.

In qualitative research, the challenge lies in maintaining objectivity when interpreting data, which typically consists of words and meanings rather than numerical values. Techniques such as reflexivity, where researchers acknowledge their own biases, and triangulation, involving the use of multiple data sources or collection methods, are employed to ensure rigor. Respondent validation, where participants review and confirm the accuracy of the study's conclusions, further strengthens the reliability of the findings. Data analysis in qualitative studies often runs parallel to data collection, enabling researchers to identify when data saturation—the point at which no new information emerges—has been reached. The analysis generally involves both inductive and deductive approaches, with themes emerging directly from the data and being compared to existing literature.

Ultimately, transparent and rigorous data analysis, whether in quantitative or qualitative research, is fundamental to producing valid, reliable, and replicable results. A detailed explanation of the analytical methods ensures that the research findings are credible and contribute meaningfully to the field.

Result

In quantitative research, results are typically presented through statistical analyses, with outcome measures such as the sample mean reported for both intervention and control groups. To determine whether observed differences are statistically significant or merely due to chance, appropriate statistical tests are applied. The P-value is used to assess the likelihood that the null hypothesis—stating there is no difference—holds true. A P-value below the predetermined threshold (commonly $P < 0.05$ or $P < 0.01$) suggests that the observed difference is statistically significant. Additionally, the inclusion of confidence intervals (CIs) provides a range within which the true population value is likely to lie, with narrower CIs indicating stronger evidence. The combined use of P-values and confidence intervals enhances the reliability of the findings and informs their potential application in practice.

In qualitative research, where the aim is to explore and interpret complex social phenomena rather than generate statistical evidence, results are typically conveyed through direct quotations or other forms of raw data that illustrate key themes. These themes and sub-themes are synthesized into core concepts, often visualized through conceptual models that represent the relationships between the findings. The process of data analysis should be rigorous, with the results clearly grounded in the data, ensuring that the conclusions drawn are logical and traceable to the original sources.

Discussion, Conclusion, and Recommendations

In quantitative research, the discussion section serves to provide a logical interpretation of the statistical findings, linking them back to the study's data while contextualizing them within the existing body of literature. The researcher should clearly address whether the study's hypothesis has been supported by the findings and explore how the results align with or deviate from prior research. Where a theoretical or conceptual framework has been employed, it is crucial to analyze how the framework relates to the results and whether the findings reinforce or challenge the theory. All interpretations and conclusions must be clearly identified and consistent with the data presented.

The significance of the findings must be carefully examined, including whether the results are both statistically significant and clinically relevant. However, this analysis should be balanced by acknowledging the study's strengths and limitations, ensuring that any potential weaknesses in the design, sampling, or analysis are clearly articulated. Another key consideration is the generalizability or external validity of the results, evaluating whether the findings can be extended beyond the specific study population to a broader context. While not all quantitative studies aim for generalizability, it is important that the researcher critically assess the study design and sampling methods to evaluate this potential.

Additionally, the researcher should consider the clinical implications of the findings, particularly in terms of how the results might inform evidence-based practice. Caution is required when proposing the practical application of the findings, as their relevance will depend on the study's specific objectives and limitations. Recommendations for future research should be clearly outlined, identifying areas that warrant further investigation and highlighting any unresolved questions raised by the study.

In qualitative research, the discussion similarly involves interpreting the findings in relation to the research question and placing them within the context of relevant literature. The researcher must critically examine how the themes and sub-themes that emerged from the data contribute to an understanding of the phenomenon under study. If a theoretical framework was employed, it is essential to explore how the framework interacts with the findings and how it deepens or expands the researcher's insights into the topic.

The significance of the qualitative findings should be discussed but balanced with a reflection on the trustworthiness of the data, including considerations of credibility, transferability, and dependability. Unlike quantitative studies, qualitative findings are not designed to be statistically generalizable. Instead, the researcher should assess the potential transferability of the results, evaluating whether the insights can be applied to similar contexts or populations to ensure the broader relevance of the study.

The practical implications of qualitative findings should also be explored, particularly in fields such as healthcare where the results may influence policy or practice. As with quantitative studies, it is important to exercise caution when suggesting practical applications, and to consider the limitations of the study in doing so. Finally, recommendations for future research should identify areas where additional studies are needed, either to deepen the understanding of the topic or to address new questions that have emerged from the data.

6.3.4 Apply

The implementation of EBP in healthcare is a multifaceted process that involves integrating the best available, current, valid, and relevant evidence into clinical decision-making [31]. This evidence comes from rigorous scientific research, clinical expertise, and updated practice guidelines that reflect the latest advancements in healthcare. Rather than focusing on generating new knowledge, EBP emphasizes the application of existing evidence to improve clinical outcomes and enhance patient care. Healthcare providers rely on credible, peer-reviewed studies to ensure that their practices are grounded in reliable and up-to-date information.

Nurses, as the largest group of healthcare professionals, play a central role in the application of EBP, directly influencing healthcare delivery and patient outcomes. Their active engagement in EBP is essential not only for improving patient care and reducing complications but also for fostering their professional growth. Through the effective application of EBP, nurses can make more informed clinical decisions, resulting in tangible benefits such as reduced pain, shorter hospital stays, lower healthcare costs, and the prevention of complications like pressure ulcers.

However, despite the clear advantages of EBP, its successful implementation in clinical settings remains challenging. The integration of EBP depends on various interrelated factors, including the characteristics of the healthcare organization, its internal and external environments, structural frameworks, and core values. Equally critical is the specific EBP focus, such as strategies aimed at reducing hospital-acquired infections, and the attitudes and perceptions of individual practitioners toward the relevance and practicality of EBP.

To address these complexities, a range of strategic approaches has been developed to support the adoption and integration of EBP. One effective strategy is to involve change advocates within the organization who can proactively tackle barriers to EBP adoption and promote a culture of continuous improvement and evidence-based decision-making. Additionally, forming multidisciplinary teams of healthcare professionals from various disciplines plays a crucial role in bridging expertise gaps and guiding the integration of EBP into organizational processes. These teams are instrumental in embedding innovative

practices that enhance the implementation of EBP, thereby transforming it into a standard of care.

Nonetheless, some critics argue that EBP's structured approach may not always account for the individualized, holistic needs of patients, questioning its flexibility and relevance in certain clinical settings. This perspective highlights the importance of applying EBP in a manner that remains adaptable to the unique context of each patient and clinical situation, ensuring that the care provided is both evidence-based and patient-centered.

The consistent application of EBP requires a dynamic interplay of organizational factors, individual practitioner engagement, and tailored strategies to address potential challenges. Establishing EBP as a standard practice involves continuous evaluation and adaptation to meet the evolving needs of both patients and the healthcare system. Fostering a supportive environment and promoting collaboration among healthcare professionals, the ultimate goal of EBP is to improve patient outcomes and elevate the overall quality of care in a sustainable and meaningful way.

6.3.4.1 Essential Apply Skills

The successful implementation of EBP requires the development of a broad range of cognitive and clinical reasoning skills, which nurses cultivate progressively over time [32]. These competencies are essential for accurately assessing patient conditions, identifying clinical problems, and locating the most reliable evidence to inform decision-making. The ultimate goal is for nurses to seamlessly organize, integrate, retrieve, and apply this knowledge within their daily clinical practice, ensuring that patient care is consistently underpinned by the most current and valid evidence.

A fundamental step in this process is the systematic organization of knowledge. Nurses must be able to structure clinical information in a manner that facilitates both its recall and its practical application in patient care scenarios. Framing knowledge around specific patient cases, nurses are better equipped to rapidly access and utilize relevant information when faced with similar clinical circumstances [33]. This process can be greatly enhanced by utilizing open-access databases and other technological tools, allowing nurses to efficiently retrieve research articles and evidence-based resources that are critical to delivering high-quality patient care.

Equally critical to EBP is the development of a strong clinical reasoning process. Beyond simply acquiring knowledge, nurses must engage in continuous, deliberate practice and seek feedback to refine their decision-making skills. Through repeated application, reflection, and self-assessment, nurses enhance their ability to translate research findings into effective clinical practice. Self-directed learning is integral to this process, enabling nurses to track their progress in understanding and applying evidence in real-world patient care settings. Passive consumption of research articles is insufficient; nurses must actively engage with the evidence and integrate it into their practice to achieve optimal patient outcomes.

Additionally, both intrinsic and extrinsic motivators are necessary for the successful adoption of EBP [9]. Internal motivation is key, as nurses must recognize the significance of EBP for their professional development and the enhancement of patient care. External incentives, often provided by healthcare organizations, also play a crucial role. These may include embedding EBP expectations within job descriptions, performance evaluations, and pathways for career advancement, all of which foster a supportive environment for evidence-based care. In specialized settings such as home healthcare, organizations that formally promote EBP through such mechanisms can significantly strengthen its integration into clinical routines.

Through the effective organization of knowledge, the cultivation of robust clinical reasoning skills, and the alignment of internal and external incentives, nurses can ensure that EBP becomes a foundational element of their daily clinical practice. This will not only improve patient outcomes but also advance the overall quality of healthcare delivery.

6.3.5 Evaluate

Evaluation is a pivotal element in the EBP process, specifically emphasized in the fifth step, which is dedicated to assessing the effectiveness and impact of implemented interventions. This step provides a systematic approach to critically analyze whether the evidence applied in clinical settings has successfully achieved its intended outcomes, guiding ongoing refinements and ensuring that healthcare practices remain evidence-informed [7].

The scope of evaluation in EBP extends far beyond the mere analysis of outcomes. It involves a comprehensive examination of PICO questions, a thorough assessment of the implementation process, and meticulous tracking of results. Such a multifaceted approach enables strategic planning and the effective design of interventions, maximizes their potential impact, and allows for mid-course adjustments to optimize clinical practices. Evaluation also serves to determine whether the implemented programs or policies have fulfilled their objectives and gathers essential data to inform the development of future EBP initiatives.

This rigorous evaluation process empowers healthcare professionals to systematically assess both the interventions and the broader context in which they are deployed. Evaluating both the intended and unintended consequences of these strategies, practitioners can make informed decisions about the relevance, effectiveness, and overall impact of EBP activities on patient care. The ultimate goal is to align these interventions with their original objectives and enhance their efficacy in improving patient outcomes.

Key principles of evaluation underscore the necessity of data-driven decision-making in healthcare, emphasizing the importance of accessible and user-friendly data for point-of-service providers [25]. Furthermore, outcome evaluation should be inherently interdisciplinary, drawing on the expertise of diverse healthcare professionals. It must also be an integral part of healthcare education, ensuring that future practitioners are well-versed in the principles of EBP and skilled in evaluating its impact on clinical practice.

Embedding these principles within both healthcare practice and education establishes a robust framework for continuous quality improvement. Through comprehensive evaluation, EBP evolves into a dynamic, adaptive process that drives sustainable enhancements in clinical decision-making, ultimately fostering high-quality patient care and promoting a culture of lifelong learning within the healthcare system [34]. This evaluative approach not only guides current practices but also shapes future strategies, ensuring that the application of evidence in healthcare is both effective and responsive to the changing needs of patients and the broader healthcare landscape.

6.4   Reviews

In the context of EBP, the use of diverse review methodologies has become indispensable for critically analyzing and synthesizing existing literature. These methodologies not only facilitate the integration of new research findings with established knowledge but also place these findings within a broader historical context, resolve inconsistencies among primary studies, and guide clinical decision-making. As the field of healthcare continues to expand, these reviews play an increasingly crucial role in building a robust evidence base that supports the implementation of EBP, enhances the quality of patient care, and directs future research endeavors.

The rapid production of research and the inherently interdisciplinary nature of healthcare present ongoing challenges for practitioners striving to stay current with the latest evidence. This situation underscores the importance of reviews as a structured and rigorous approach to the collection, analysis, and synthesis of relevant studies. Such scholarly endeavors are essential for uncovering the current state of knowledge, identifying critical gaps, justifying new investigations, and establishing a framework for research objectives, questions, and methodologies. This meticulous review process not only validates existing clinical practices but also drives innovation and continuous improvement in

healthcare strategies. Providing a cohesive synthesis of data from multiple studies, reviews play a pivotal role in optimizing clinical decision-making, enhancing patient outcomes, and advancing healthcare research, thereby contributing to the evolution of evidence-based interventions and the sustained progress of the healthcare sector.

The growing acknowledgment of the importance of reviews has led to the development of a broader range of review types across nursing and other disciplines. Concurrently, the field of evidence synthesis has experienced significant growth and transformation. The increasing need to integrate and analyze diverse forms of evidence has driven the creation of innovative methodologies designed to rigorously synthesize data and address complex questions relevant to policymakers, researchers, and practitioners. In their 2009 study, Grant and Booth identified 14 distinct types of review methods [35]. This array of evidence synthesis methods expanded to 25 by 2016 [36], and further evolved to encompass 48 different review types by 2019 [37]. These developments underscore the dynamic progression and refinement of approaches in the domain of evidence synthesis.

6.4.1   Major Type of Review

Review articles come in various forms, each designed to serve specific research purposes and questions. The nine major types of reviews include: Umbrella Review, Systematic Review with Meta-Analysis, Systematic Review with Meta-Synthesis, Systematic Review, Rapid Review, Scoping Review, Integrative Review, Critical Review, and Literature Review. Each of these review types employs distinct methodologies for synthesizing research evidence, enabling researchers to choose the most suitable approach to address their specific research questions and objectives Table 6.5.

6.4.1.1 Umbrella Review
An Umbrella Review, also referred to as an "overview," "review of reviews," or "meta-

Table 6.5 Comparison of major types of reviews

Review type	Description	Strengths	Weaknesses
Umbrella review	Compiles evidence from multiple systematic reviews into a cohesive document, focusing on broad conditions or problems	Provides a comprehensive summary of multiple reviews; highest level of synthesis; captures overarching patterns	Depends on existing systematic reviews; limited applicability in areas lacking sufficient reviews
Systematic review with meta-analysis	Combines structured methodology of a systematic review with statistical aggregation of data to derive an accurate effect size	Enhances power and precision; transforms diverse findings into cohesive evidence; reliable for guiding decisions	Requires homogeneous data; risk of bias if studies are too varied ("apples and oranges" problem)
Systematic review with meta-synthesis	Integrates systematic review methods with interpretative synthesis of qualitative studies to uncover deeper insights	Offers a richer understanding of qualitative data; develops new theories and frameworks; valuable in complex areas	Subjective interpretation; challenges in integrating diverse qualitative methods and maintaining consistency
Systematic review	Uses a structured approach to search, appraise, and synthesize research evidence to generate a comprehensive summary	Delivers unbiased and detailed analysis; includes quantitative, qualitative, and mixed-method research	Traditionally focused on specific study designs, limiting exploration of broader questions or mechanisms
Rapid review	A streamlined review process designed for quick decision-making, often used to meet urgent policy or practice needs	Balances rigor and efficiency; accelerates evidence synthesis; useful for timely insights	Risk of bias due to limited search strategies and appraisal; may overlook relevant studies or emphasize lower-quality research
Scoping review	Maps the size, scope, and nature of existing research literature to provide a preliminary overview of a topic	Identifies research gaps; helps determine if a full systematic review is needed; adaptable to the scope of evidence	Lacks critical appraisal; vulnerable to bias; does not provide concrete recommendations for practice or policy
Integrative review	Synthesizes qualitative and quantitative data from diverse studies to present a broader understanding of a topic	Combines varied perspectives; bridges empirical data with theoretical insights; valuable for holistic evidence	Complexity in integrating different methodologies; risk of inconsistencies and potential biases in synthesis
Critical review	Analyses and synthesizes diverse sources to develop new models or theories beyond established frameworks	Offers fresh insights; evaluates existing knowledge critically; drives theoretical development	Lacks structured search and synthesis; interpretative nature may lead to subjectivity and limited methodological rigor
Literature review (narrative/state-of-the-art)	Examines and summarizes existing literature to provide an overview of the current state of knowledge	Consolidates knowledge; identifies gaps and trends; guides future research	Potential bias due to non-systematic approach; may overemphasize studies aligning with the author's perspective

review," has emerged as a crucial approach in response to the growing number of systematic reviews [38]. As the volume of systematic reviews continues to expand, the need for these comprehensive reviews has increased, offering a means to synthesize findings from multiple reviews that focus on specific research questions. An Umbrella Review compiles evidence from various systematic reviews into a single, cohesive document, particularly useful when these reviews explore a broad condition or problem with multiple poten-

tial interventions. This review type now stands at the **top of the evidence hierarchy**, representing the highest level of synthesis by integrating data from numerous systematic reviews [12].

The key strength of Umbrella Reviews lies in their ability to deliver a comprehensive and accessible summary of multiple reviews, serving as a valuable resource for understanding the overall landscape of evidence on a particular topic. They effectively address the challenge researchers' face when deciding whether to "lump" diverse interventions into a broader analysis, which may lead to a loss of detail, or "split" them into more focused reviews that could fragment the bigger picture [39]. Through the synthesis of data from multiple reviews into a coherent narrative, Umbrella Reviews offer a balanced approach that captures overarching patterns and insights across various studies.

However, the primary limitation of Umbrella Reviews is their reliance on the existence of narrower, component reviews. Without these foundational systematic reviews, producing a thorough Umbrella Review becomes challenging, limiting its applicability in areas where such reviews are scarce. Despite this dependency, Umbrella Reviews are highly effective in synthesizing evidence across diverse domains, such as health library outreach services, to identify the conditions under which one intervention may be more favorable than another. This capacity to integrate and interpret extensive data sets makes Umbrella Reviews an invaluable tool for guiding decision-making and advancing knowledge in complex fields.

6.4.1.2 Systematic Review with Meta-analysis

A Systematic Review with Meta-analysis represents a rigorous approach to synthesizing research evidence, combining the structured methodology of a systematic review with the statistical precision of meta-analysis. This comprehensive method systematically identifies, appraises, and integrates relevant studies, followed by a meta-analytic process that quantitatively aggregates their results [40]. The aim is to derive a more accurate estimate of the overall effect size, thereby enhancing the robustness and reliability of the conclusions drawn from the evidence.

The principal strength of a meta-analysis lies in its capacity to consolidate data from multiple studies, even when individual studies have limited sample sizes or inconclusive findings. The statistical combination of these results enhances the overall power and precision of the analysis, providing a clearer understanding of the effectiveness of interventions or treatments. This method transforms disparate research findings into a cohesive body of evidence, serving as a critical resource for clinicians, policymakers, and researchers who require the most reliable data to guide decision-making and inform practice.

However, the validity of a meta-analysis is inherently linked to the quality and homogeneity of the included studies. One of the central challenges is the risk of integrating heterogeneous studies, often referred to as the issue of combining "apples and oranges," where differences in study designs, populations, or outcome measures can undermine the credibility of the findings [41]. To mitigate this risk, careful selection criteria and rigorous evaluation are essential to ensure that only comparable studies are included. Executed with precision, a systematic review with meta-analysis stands as one of the highest tiers of evidence in research, offering a robust framework for advancing evidence-based practice and guiding future investigations.

6.4.1.3 Systematic Review with Meta-Synthesis

A systematic review with meta-synthesis represents a rigorous approach in qualitative research, integrating the structured methodology of systematic review with the interpretative depth of meta-synthesis. This method involves systematically identifying, appraising, and synthesizing findings from qualitative studies to uncover underlying themes, patterns, and insights that contribute to a comprehensive understanding of complex phenomena. Unlike quantitative meta-analysis, which relies on statistical aggregation, a meta-synthesis focuses on interpreting and integrating data from diverse qualitative studies to develop new theories or conceptual frameworks.

The strength of a meta-synthesis lies in its ability to integrate disparate qualitative data, offering a richer understanding of complex issues, particularly in fields like healthcare, education, and social sciences, where human experiences and perspectives are central [42]. However, challenges include the diversity of qualitative methods and the subjective nature of interpretation, which can affect the consistency of findings.

Despite these challenges, a well-conducted meta-synthesis is a powerful tool that enhances the understanding of qualitative data and generates new theoretical insights. It plays a crucial role in bridging the gap between individual study findings and broader theoretical frameworks, guiding evidence-based decision-making in research and practice.

6.4.1.4 Systematic Review

A systematic review is a well-established method in research, meticulously designed to search, appraise, and synthesize evidence in a structured manner. It adheres to rigorous guidelines, such as those provided by the Cochrane Collaboration and the Agency for Healthcare Research and Quality (AHRQ), ensuring that its methods are transparent and replicable. The aim of a systematic review is to produce a comprehensive synthesis of the existing knowledge base, facilitating the replication of its findings and enhancing the reliability of the conclusions drawn.

The key strength of systematic reviews lies in their capacity to integrate all relevant evidence on a particular topic, delivering a detailed and unbiased overview. In recent years, initiatives by organizations like the Campbell Collaboration and the Cochrane Qualitative Methods Group have significantly broadened the scope of these reviews. This evolution has led to the inclusion of diverse study designs, incorporating quantitative, qualitative, and mixed-method research [43]. Such inclusivity has enriched the applicability and relevance of Systematic Reviews across a wider range of disciplines, enabling a more holistic understanding of complex research questions.

Systematic reviews are invaluable tools in synthesizing research evidence, yet they are not without limitations. Their rigorous inclusion criteria often lead to the exclusion of studies that do not meet specific methodological standards, thereby narrowing the scope and potentially omitting relevant data. The validity of a systematic review heavily depends on the quality of the included studies; any methodological flaws in these studies can compromise the reliability of the review's conclusions [44]. Additionally, publication bias is a significant concern, as systematic reviews primarily draw upon published studies, which can lead to an overemphasis on positive outcomes. The extensive time required to conduct systematic reviews can result in findings that may no longer be current by the time of publication. Furthermore, systematic reviews typically focus on assessing the effectiveness of interventions, often neglecting the exploration of underlying mechanisms or contextual factors that could influence outcomes. Expanding the range of included study designs and integrating both quantitative and qualitative data could enhance the comprehensiveness and applicability of systematic reviews in guiding evidence-based practice.

6.4.1.5 Rapid Review

A Rapid Review is an evidence synthesis approach designed to deliver timely insights, particularly for policymakers requiring quick decision support. Initially seen as a compromise to accommodate the **fast-paced** demands of policy development, Rapid Reviews have since evolved into formal Rapid Evidence Assessments. These assessments utilize systematic review methods to critically appraise existing research, offering concise evaluations of what is already known about specific policy or practice issues [45].

The strength of Rapid Reviews lies in their ability to balance rigor with efficiency. Refining research questions, simplifying search strategies, limiting gray literature, and conducting basic quality assessments accelerate the review process while maintaining systematic principles [45]. This pragmatic approach allows for faster evidence synthesis, essential for responsive decision-making.

However, the speed of Rapid Reviews can increase the risk of bias, as limited searches and appraisals may overlook relevant studies or emphasize lower-quality research [46]. Documenting methodological limitations is crucial to ensure transparency and mitigate these biases. Despite their limitations, Rapid Reviews play a critical role in evidence-based policymaking, offering a structured yet flexible approach to meet urgent information needs.

6.4.1.6 Scoping Review

A Scoping Review, also known as a Mapping Review, offers a preliminary assessment of the size and scope of existing research literature, with the aim of mapping the nature and extent of the available evidence, including ongoing studies [47]. This type of review is a valuable tool for gaining a broad understanding of a research topic, providing insights into the overall landscape of knowledge and highlighting areas that require further exploration.

One of the key strengths of Scoping Reviews is their ability to inform policymakers and researchers about the feasibility of conducting a full systematic review. They share core principles with systematic reviews, such as a commitment to systematic, transparent, and replicable methods, which help ensure a structured approach to the literature [47].

However, Scoping Reviews have inherent limitations that prevent them from serving as definitive evidence sources. Their reduced methodological rigor and the absence of a formal quality assessment make them vulnerable to bias, as they tend to focus on the existence of studies rather than their quality. This lack of critical appraisal limits their ability to provide concrete recommendations for policy or practice [48]. Nonetheless, Scoping Reviews play an essential role in identifying research gaps and shaping future research agendas, acting as a foundational step toward more comprehensive and in-depth evidence syntheses.

6.4.1.7 Integrative Review

An Integrative Review, also known as an "Integrative Literature Review" or "Integrative Synthesis," is a comprehensive approach that synthesizes qualitative and quantitative data from diverse empirical and theoretical studies [25]. This method uniquely integrates various research designs to provide a broader understanding of complex phenomena, making it a crucial tool in evidence-based nursing and related fields. Its primary goal is to generate insights, guide clinical practice, inform research directions, and shape policy development.

The strength of an Integrative Review lies in its ability to present a holistic view of evidence by incorporating findings from a range of study designs, offering deeper insights into multifaceted issues in healthcare. It effectively bridges the gap between empirical research and theoretical frameworks, enhancing decision-making and advancing knowledge in the field. However, challenges arise in integrating diverse methodologies, which can impact rigor and consistency, leading to potential biases. The complexity of synthesizing heterogeneous data highlights the need for more structured and transparent guidelines. Despite these limitations, integrative reviews remain essential for advancing evidence-based practice by offering comprehensive perspectives that inform both clinical and policy decisions.

6.4.1.8 Critical Review

A Critical Review serves to demonstrate a comprehensive exploration of the literature, emphasizing critical analysis and conceptual innovation. Rather than merely describing existing studies, it synthesizes material from diverse sources, often resulting in a hypothesis or model that extends beyond established frameworks [49]. This type of review aims to reinterpret existing data or blend various theories to present new perspectives.

The true strength of a Critical Review lies in its ability to evaluate existing knowledge critically, offering fresh insights that can resolve competing ideas and drive future theoretical development. It allows for a systematic reassessment of existing concepts, providing a foundation for further conceptual advancements. However, Critical Reviews often lack the structured approach seen in systematic reviews, as they do not require detailed methods of search, synthesis, or analysis. The focus is on conceptual contributions rather than strict methodological rigor, making the interpretative nature of these reviews subjective. As a result, a Critical Review serves as a starting point for further investigation, offering a conceptual basis for future research rather than a definitive conclusion.

6.4.1.9 Literature Review (Narrative or State-of-the-Art Review)

A Literature Review, also known as a Narrative Review or State-of-the-Art Review, examines published materials to provide a comprehensive overview of the current state of knowledge on a specific subject [50]. It evaluates sources like peer-reviewed articles, focusing on credible content to ensure reliability. The review process involves identifying relevant studies, selecting appropriate materials, and synthesizing findings through textual, tabular, or graphical formats, followed by a critical analysis of their contributions to the field.

The strength of a Literature Review lies in its ability to consolidate knowledge, build on prior research, and identify gaps within the literature, guiding future research and preventing duplication of efforts. It creates a coherent narrative that highlights established findings, shaping the direction of scholarly inquiry. However, Literature Reviews may lack a systematic approach, leading to potential bias by omitting significant works or emphasizing studies that align with the author's perspective. While indispensable for summarizing knowledge, they must be conducted with objectivity and critical assessment to ensure a balanced representation of the research landscape.

6.4.2 Selecting Type of Review

Selecting the most appropriate type of review for a research project is a multifaceted decision that hinges on several critical factors, including the purpose of the research question, the composition and expertise of the research team, and the time available to conduct the study. Equally important is the consideration of how the chosen review type will contribute to the broader advancement of knowledge within the discipline.

In scenarios where a research team is adequately sized, possesses diverse expertise, and has sufficient time to conduct a systematic review, but the initial search of the literature yields limited information on the specific question, it may be more effective to broaden the focus and under-

take a scoping review. This approach allows for a more comprehensive exploration of the topic while remaining adaptable to the scope of available evidence. Conversely, if the research question is broad and the team faces limitations in expanding its size or available time, a narrative literature review may be a more suitable and pragmatic choice.

Conducting a systematic review can present challenges if the results from the included studies are too heterogeneous to be effectively synthesized; under these circumstances, a meta-analysis or meta-synthesis may not be feasible due to the difficulty in combining varied findings [23]. In such situations, a critical or integrative review may offer a more suitable approach for evaluating the evidence. Additionally, if the research question involves a novel treatment, device, or educational approach, and the team possesses sufficient expertise but operates under time constraints, a rapid review might be the most appropriate strategy to provide timely, evidence-based insights [40].

Ultimately, aligning the type of literature review with the specific objectives of the research project, the resources available, and the potential impact on the field ensures that the chosen approach maximizes both the quality of the analysis and its contribution to the scientific community. This careful alignment not only enhances the rigor and relevance of the review but also supports the broader goals of knowledge synthesis and evidence-based practice within the discipline.

6.5 Barriers to Evidence-based Practice

The disparity in healthcare performance is often attributed to the gap between knowledge generation and its application in clinical practice. Barriers to the implementation of EBP are frequently identified as modifiable factors that, when addressed, can significantly enhance the organizational and environmental context, as well as improve educational strategies [51, 52]. A deeper understanding of these barriers is essential, as it holds the potential to shift attitudes and beliefs about EBP, creating a more supportive framework for its integration into healthcare settings.

Despite the proven benefits of EBP in elevating the quality of care and improving patient outcomes, numerous challenges persist in its adoption and implementation. The literature highlights key obstacles such as limited time, lack of knowledge and expertise, insufficient medical resources, financial limitations, and negative attitudes toward EBP [53]. Overcoming these barriers is crucial to bridging the gap between research and practice, thereby ensuring that healthcare delivery is guided by the most current and effective evidence available. Addressing these challenges will not only strengthen the foundation for EBP but also pave the way for a more robust and responsive healthcare system.

6.5.1   Organizational Barriers

Organizational barriers are among the most significant obstacles to implementing EBP in nursing. Many nurses face challenges such as limited time, inadequate access to essential resources, and a lack of institutional support, which collectively hinder the consistent adoption of EBP in clinical settings [54]. Despite national initiatives aimed at promoting EBP within healthcare, its widespread implementation remains inconsistent in nursing environments [51, 55]. Although the benefits of EBP are well-documented, it has yet to be fully embraced as a standard of care across the profession.

Key organizational factors that impede EBP integration include insufficient time for sourcing, critically evaluating, and applying evidence-based interventions as well as a lack of authority for nurses to modify existing care practices [56]. Often, nurses operate within a workplace culture resistant to innovation, where traditional protocols and practices dominate over the adoption of new evidence-based strategies. Overcoming these organizational barriers necessitates the development of a supportive culture that empow-

ers nurses, ensures access to necessary resources, and prioritizes continuous improvement and innovation in clinical practice [57]. Establishing such a culture is essential for embedding EBP into the everyday practice of nursing and enhancing patient outcomes.

6.5.2   Educational Barriers

Educational barriers represent a critical challenge in the integration of EBP within nursing. Deficiencies in language proficiency, limited research skills, and inadequate training in statistical methods significantly impede nurses' ability to interpret and apply research findings in clinical settings [58]. Current nursing education programs often fall short in equipping practitioners with the comprehensive knowledge and skills necessary for effective EBP implementation, resulting in substantial gaps in their capacity to critically evaluate and utilize evidence [57].

Although various educational initiatives have been developed to enhance nurses' understanding of EBP principles, these efforts alone are insufficient for the seamless incorporation of EBP into everyday practice. To facilitate the widespread adoption of EBP, nursing education must place greater emphasis on cultivating critical thinking abilities and strengthening research evaluation skills [59]. Focusing on these competencies, educational programs can better prepare nurses to make informed clinical decisions that are grounded in the most up-to-date and robust evidence available. This approach is essential for advancing the quality of patient care and ensuring that nursing practice evolves in alignment with the latest scientific developments.

6.5.3   Individual Barriers

Individual barriers present a significant challenge to the adoption of EBP among nurses. A lack of essential knowledge, skills, and awareness related to EBP is a prevalent issue, with many nurses experiencing difficulty in understanding and applying research findings [60]. This struggle often stems from limited critical appraisal abilities and an unfamiliarity with statistical concepts. Additionally, personal factors, such as low confidence in their ability to assess research and a perception that their EBP skills are insufficient, further impede the integration of evidence-based approaches into clinical practice [61].

High workloads and time constraints also play a substantial role in discouraging nurses from actively seeking or incorporating evidence-based information into their routines [62]. In contrast, nurses with better access to resources, such as electronic databases, professional guidelines, and educational tools, are more likely to effectively utilize EBP in their decision-making processes [63]. Overcoming these individual barriers requires a focused effort to develop the necessary competencies and self-assurance among nurses, fostering a culture that prioritizes continuous learning and the consistent application of evidence-based care [57].This approach is crucial to empowering nurses to deliver high-quality, research-informed care in diverse clinical environments.

6.5.4 Research-related Barriers

Research-related barriers pose significant challenges to the implementation of EBP in nursing. A primary obstacle is the scarcity of high-quality, clinically relevant research that directly addresses the specific needs of nursing practice [64]. Even when relevant evidence is available, its integration into clinical settings is often slow due to inefficient knowledge translation and dissemination processes, which limit its practical application [65].

Nurses frequently encounter difficulties in accessing and interpreting research due to the complexity of its presentation and the technical language used in scholarly articles [66]. Without adequate support, these challenges can hinder the effective utilization of evidence. Furthermore, contextual variations across different clinical settings can lead to conflicting interpretations of research findings, complicating nurses' efforts to

identify the most appropriate course of action for patient care.

To address these research-related barriers, efforts must be directed toward enhancing the quality, clarity, and accessibility of evidence as well as strengthening strategies for knowledge translation to ensure that research findings are readily applicable to nursing practice [10]. Significant investment in nursing-specific resources, such as specialized research databases, targeted training in evidence appraisal, and robust institutional support, is essential. Establishing an environment that equips nurses with the essential time, tools, and resources to engage in evidence-based practice will allow the healthcare system to enhance patient outcomes and develop a more empowered and research-informed nursing workforce.

References

1. Cochrane A. Effectiveness and efficiency: random reflections on health services [Internet]. London: Nuffield Trust; 1972 [cited 2024 Sep 18]. https://www.nuffieldtrust.org.uk/research/effectiveness-and-efficiency-random-reflections-on-health-services.
2. Cochrane. Cochrane trusted evidence. Informed decisions. Better health [Internet]; 2024 [cited 2024 Sep 18]. https://www.cochrane.org/about-us.
3. Sackett DL, Rosenberg WMC, Gray JAM, Haynes RB, Richardson WS. Evidence based medicine: what it is and what it isn't. BMJ. 1996;312(7023):71–2.
4. Melnyk BM, Fineout-Overholt E. Making the case for evidence-based practice and cultivating a spirit of inquiry. Evidence-based practice in nursing & healthcare: a guide to best practice. 2nd ed. Philadelphia: Wolters Kluwer; 2023. p. 1–24.
5. ICN. Closing the gap: from evidence to action. Geneva: International Council of Nurses; 2012. p. 1–59.
6. Ingersoll GL. Evidence-based nursing: what it is and what it isn't. Nurs Outlook. 2000;48(4):151–2.
7. Law M, MacDermid JC. Introduction to evidence-based practice. In: Law M, MacDermid JC, editors. Evidence-based rehabilitation. 3rd ed. New York: Routledge; 2024.
8. Schmidt NA, Brown JM. What is evidence-based practice? In: Schmider NA, Brown JM, editors. Evidence-based practice for nurses: appraisal and application of research with navigate advantage access. Burlington: Jones & Bartlett Learning; 2024.
9. Godshall M. Fast facts for evidence-based practice in nursing. Berlin: Springer; 2024.

10. Connor L, Dean J, McNett M, Tydings DM, Shrout A, Gorsuch PF, et al. Evidence-based practice improves patient outcomes and healthcare system return on investment: findings from a scoping review. Worldviews Evid-Based Nurs. 2023;20(1):6–15.

11. Dykes PC, Curtin-Bowen M, Lipsitz S, Franz C, Adelman J, Adkison L, et al. Cost of inpatient falls and cost-benefit analysis of implementation of an evidence-based fall prevention program. JAMA Health Forum. 2023;4(1):e225125.

12. Choi GJ, Kang H. Introduction to umbrella reviews as a useful evidence-based practice. J Lipid Atheroscler. 2023;12(1):3–11.

13. White KM. The science of translation and major frameworks. In: White KM, Dudley-Brown S, Terhaar MF, editors. Translation of evidence into nursing and healthcare. Berlin: Springer; 2024.

14. Dusin J, Melanson A, Mische-Lawson L. Evidence-based practice models and frameworks in the healthcare setting: a scoping review. BMJ Open. 2023;13(5):e071188.

15. Iowa Model Collaborative, Buckwalter KC, Cullen L, Hanrahan K, Kleiber C, McCarthy AM, et al. Iowa model of evidence-based practice: revisions and validation. Worldviews Evid-Based Nurs. 2017;14(3):175–82.

16. Newhouse RP, Dearholt S, Poe S, Pugh LC, White KM. Organizational change strategies for evidence-based practice. J Nurs Adm. 2007;37(12):552–7.

17. Kring DL. Clinical nurse specialist practice domains and evidence-based practice competencies: a matrix of influence. Clin Nurse Spec. 2008;22(4):179–83.

18. Melnyk BM. Achieving a high-reliability organization through implementation of the ARCC model for systemwide sustainability of evidence-based practice. Nurs Adm Q. 2012;36(2):127–35.

19. Jordan Z, Lockwood C, Munn Z, Aromataris E. The updated Joanna Briggs institute model of evidence-based healthcare. Int J Evid Based Healthc. 2019;17(1):58–71.

20. Hosseini M-S, Jahanshahlou F, Akbarzadeh MA, Zarei M, Vaez-Gharamaleki Y. Formulating research questions for evidence-based studies. J Med Surg Public Health. 2024;2:100046.

21. Willis LD. Formulating the research question and framing the hypothesis. Respir Care. 2023;68(8):1180–5.

22. Hays D, Milner KA, Farus-Brown S, Zonsius MC, Fineout-Overholt E. Clinical inquiry and problem identification. Am J Nurs. 2024;124(5):38.

23. Mancin S, Sguanci M, Anastasi G, Godino L, Lo Cascio A, Morenghi E, et al. A methodological framework for rigorous systematic reviews: tailoring comprehensive analyses to clinicians and healthcare professionals. Methods. 2024;225:38–43.

24. McKenzie J, Brennan SE, Ryan RE, Thomson HJ, Johnston RV, Thomas J. Chapter 3: Defining the criteria for including studies and how they will be grouped for the synthesis [last updated August 2023]. In: JPT H, Thomas J, Chandler J, Cumpston M, Li T, Page MJ, et al., editors. Cochrane handbook for systematic reviews of interventions version 6.5. Cochrane [Internet]. Wiley; 2024. [cited 2024 Oct 10]. www.training.cochrane.org/handbook.

25. Bettany-Saltikov J, McSherry R. How to do a systematic literature review in nursing: a step-by-step guide. 3rd ed. Maidenhead: McGraw-Hill Education; 2024.

26. Komukai K, Sugita S, Fujimoto S. Publication bias and selective outcome reporting in randomized controlled trials related to rehabilitation: a literature review. Arch Phys Med Rehabil. 2024;105(1):150–6.

27. Rojas-Saunero LP, Glymour MM, Mayeda ER. Selection bias in health research: quantifying, eliminating, or exacerbating health disparities? Curr Epidemiol Rep. 2024;11(1):63–72.

28. Konno K, Gibbons J, Lewis R, Pullin AS. Potential types of bias when estimating causal effects in environmental research and how to interpret them. Environ Evid. 2024;13(1):1.

29. Grove SK, Gray JR. Understanding nursing research: building an evidence-based practice. Amsterdam: Elsevier; 2022.

30. CASP. Critical Appraisal Skills Programme [Internet]; 2024 [cited 2024 Oct 10]. https://casp-uk.net.

31. Stanik-Hutt J. Translation of evidence to improve clinical outcome. In: White KM, Dudley-Brown S, Terhaar MF, editors. Translation of evidence into nursing and healthcare. Berlin: Springer; 2024.

32. Hollowood L, Moorley C. Embracing diversity in nursing research: essential tips. Evidence-based nursing [Internet]. Royal College of Nursing; 30 Aug 2024 [cited 2024 Oct 10]. https://ebn.bmj.com/content/early/2024/08/30/ebnurs-2024-104183.

33. Spain S. Appraising the evidence to determine the best practices. In: Schmider NA, Brown JM, editors. Evidence-based practice for nurses: appraisal and application of research with navigate advantage access. Burington: Jones & Bartlett Learning; 2024.

34. While K. Translation of evidence for improving safety and quality. In: White KM, Dudley-Brown S, Terhaar MF, editors. Translation of evidence into nursing and healthcare. Berlin: Springer; 2024.

35. Grant MJ, Booth A. A typology of reviews: an analysis of 14 review types and associated methodologies. Health Inf Libr J. 2009;26(2):91–108.

36. Tricco AC, Soobiah C, Antony J, Cogo E, MacDonald H, Lillie E, et al. A scoping review identifies multiple emerging knowledge synthesis methods, but few studies operationalize the method. J Clin Epidemiol. 2016;73:19–28.

37. Sutton A, Clowes M, Preston L, Booth A. Meeting the review family: exploring review types and associated information retrieval requirements. Health Info Libr J. 2019;36(3):202–22.

38. Pollock M, Fernandes RM, Becker LA, Pieper D, Butler LD. Chapter V: Overviews of reviews. In: Higgins JP, Thomas J, Chandel J, Cumpston M, Li T, Page M, et al., editors. Cochrane handbook for systematic reviews of interventions 6.3 [Internet]. 2nd

ed. Chichester: Wiley; 2024. www.training.cochrane.org/handbook.

39. Belbasis L, Bellou V, Ioannidis JPA. Conducting umbrella reviews. bmjmed [internet]. BMJ Publishing; 22 Nov 2022 [cited 2024 Oct 10];1(1). https://bmj-medicine.bmj.com/content/1/1/e000071.

40. Mayo-Wilson E, Qureshi R, Li T. Conducting separate reviews of benefits and harms could improve systematic reviews and meta-analyses. Syst Rev. 2023;12(1):67.

41. Lee KS, Prevedello DM. Systematic reviews and meta-analyses in neurosurgery part II: a guide to designing the protocol. Neurosurg Rev. 2024;47(1):360.

42. Glisic M, Raguindin PF, Gemperli A, Taneri PE, Salvador DJ, Voortman T, et al. A 7-step guideline for qualitative synthesis and meta-analysis of observational studies in health sciences. Public Health Rev. 2023;44:1605454.

43. Nelson HD. Systematic reviews. In: Nelson HD, editor. Systematic reviews to answer health care questions. Philadelphia: Lippincott Williams & Wilkins; 2024.

44. Kolaski K, Logan LR, Ioannidis JPA. Guidance to best tools and practices for systematic reviews. Syst Rev. 2023;12(1):96.

45. Garritty C, Hamel C, Trivella M, Gartlehner G, Nussbaumer-Streit B, Devane D, et al. Updated recommendations for the Cochrane rapid review methods guidance for rapid reviews of effectiveness. BMJ. 2024;384:e076335.

46. Gartlehner G, Nussbaumer-Streit B, Devane D, Kahwati L, Viswanathan M, King VJ, et al. Rapid reviews methods series: guidance on assessing the certainty of evidence. BMJ Evid Based Med. 2024;29(1):50–4.

47. Khalil H, Campbell F, Danial K, Pollock D, Munn Z, Welsh V, et al. Advancing the methodology of mapping reviews: a scoping review. Res Synth Methods. 2024;15(3):384–97.

48. Campbell F, Tricco AC, Munn Z, Pollock D, Saran A, Sutton A, et al. Mapping reviews, scoping reviews, and evidence and gap maps (EGMs): the same but different— the "Big Picture" review family. Syst Rev. 2023;12(1):45.

49. Davies M. Writing critical reviews: a step-by-step guide. In: Davies M, editor. Study skills for international postgraduates. 2nd ed. New York: Bloomsbury Academic; 2022. p. 194–207.

50. Buchholz SW, Dickins KA. Literature review and synthesis typology. In: Buchholz SW, Dickins KA, editors. Literature review and synthesis: a guide for nurses and other healthcare professionals. Springer; 2023.

51. Huo M, Qin H, Zhou X, Li J, Zhao B, Li Y. Impact of an organizational climate for evidence-based practice on evidence-based practice behaviour among nurses: mediating effects of competence, work control, and intention for evidence-based practice implementation. J Nurs Manag. 2024;2024(1):5972218.

52. Mohamed RA, Alhujaily M, Ahmed FA, Nouh WG, Almowafy AA. Nurses' experiences and perspectives regarding evidence-based practice implementation in healthcare context: a qualitative study. Nurs Open. 2024;11(1):e2080.

53. Furtado L, Coelho F, Mendonça N, Soares H, Gomes L, Sousa JP, et al. Exploring professional practice environments and organisational context factors affecting nurses' adoption of evidence-based practice: a scoping review. Healthcare. 2024;12(2):245.

54. Torres C, Mendes F, Duarte AM, Vilaça S, Barbieri-Figueiredo M, do C. Implementation of evidence-based practice in paediatric nursing care: facilitators and barriers. Collegian. 2024;31(5):342–7.

55. Horning MA, Taylor-Pearson ZA. Nurse leaders as influencers of knowledge to practice. Worldviews Evid-Based Nurs. 2024;21(3):230–3.

56. Zhang Y, Guo Z, Xu S, Yao M, Feng X, Lan M, et al. Facilitating evidence-based practice among nurses in a tertiary general hospital: a six-year practice of an implementation strategy informed by the i-PARIHS framework. J Nurs Manag. 2024;2024(1):8855667.

57. Paul J. Transitioning evidence to practice. In: Schmidt NA, Brown JM, editors. Evidence-based practice for nurses: appraisal and application of research with navigate advantage access. Burlington: Jones & Bartlett Learning; 2024.

58. Nielsen LD, Castano FM, Jørgensen RB, Ramachandran A, Egebæk HK, Noe BB. Teaching evidence-based practice to undergraduate healthcare students educators' knowledge, skills, attitudes, current practice, perceived barriers, and facilitators: a Danish cross-sectional study. Nurse Educ Today. 2024;133:106082.

59. Vaajoki A, Kvist T, Kulmala M, Tervo-Heikkinen T. Systematic education has a positive impact on nurses' evidence-based practice: intervention study results. Nurse Educ Today. 2023;120:105597.

60. Smith S, Johnson G. A systematic review of the barriers, enablers and strategies to embedding translational research within the public hospital system focusing on nursing and allied health professions. PLoS One. 2023;18(2):e0281819.

61. Sampson M, Knupp A, Chignolli H, Dhakal K, Bulkowski K, Perdue J, et al. Strategies for incorporating evidence-based practice into nurse residency programs: a scoping review. Worldviews Evid-Based Nurs. 2024;21(4):407–14.

62. Arsenault Knudsen ÉN, Mundt MP, Steege LM. Describing nurses' communication about evidence-based practice change: a social network analysis of hospital nurses. Worldviews Evid-Based Nurs. 2024;21(2):128–36.

63. Fineout-Overholt E, Hays D, Farus-Brown S, Zonsius MC, Milner KA. Removing persistent barriers to systematic searching. Am J Nurs. 2024;124(7):40.

64. Furuki H, Sonoda N, Morimoto A. Factors related to the knowledge and skills of evidence-based prac-

tice among nurses worldwide: a scoping review. Worldviews Evid-Based Nurs. 2023;20(1):16–26.

65. Hosseini-Moghaddam F, Mohammadpour A, Bahri N, Mojalli M. Nursing managers' perspectives on facilitators of and barriers to evidence-based practice: a cross-sectional study. Nurs Open. 2023;10(9):6237–47.

66. Adombire S, Baiden D, Puts M, Puchalski Ritchie LM, Ani-Amponsah M, Cranley L. Knowledge, skills, attitudes, beliefs, and implementation of evidence-based practice among nurses in low- and middle-income countries: a scoping review. Worldviews Evid-Based Nurs. 2024;21(5):542–53.